HAIR
magic

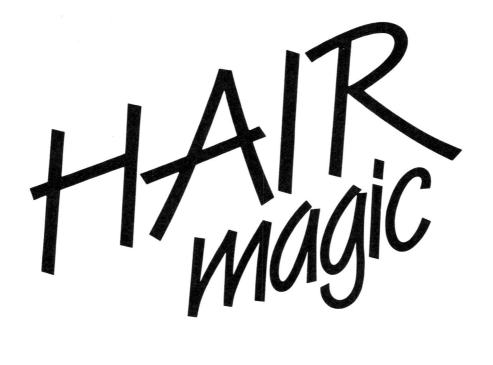

HAIR magic

A COMPLETE GUIDE TO CUTTING, STYLING, TINTING AND COLOURING YOUR HAIR
AT HOME AND IN THE SALON

Marion Mathews and Renske Mann

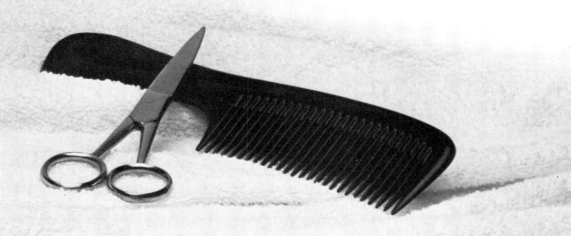

Macdonald

A Macdonald BOOK

© Swallow Publishing Limited 1984.

First published in Great Britain in 1984
by Macdonald & Co (Publishers) Ltd
London & Sydney

A member of BPCC plc

British Library Cataloguing in Publication Data

Mathews, Marion
 Hair magic.
 1. Hair – Care and hygiene
 I. Title   II. Mann, Renske
 646.7'24   RL91
 ISBN 0-356-10499 0

Typeset in Helvetica Light by
Wagstaff Design Associates

Origination by
John Swain and Son Ltd

Printed and bound in Spain by
Mateu Cromo
Artes Graficas, SA,
Madrid

Conceived and produced by
Swallow Publishing Limited
32 Hermes Street, London N1

Editor Loulou Brown
Editorial assistant Angie Doran
Hairdressing consultant Christine Harvey
Art director David Young
Designer Glynis Edwards
Assistant designer Lynn Hector
Design assistant Susan Brinkhurst
Studio Del and co
Step-by-step illustrator Coral Mula
Picture research Liz Eddison

All statements in this book giving information and advice are believed to
be true and accurate at the time of going to press, but neither the authors
nor the publishers can accept legal responsibility for errors or
omissions.

Macdonald & Co (Publishers) Ltd
Maxwell House
74 Worship Street
London EC2A 2EN

Contents

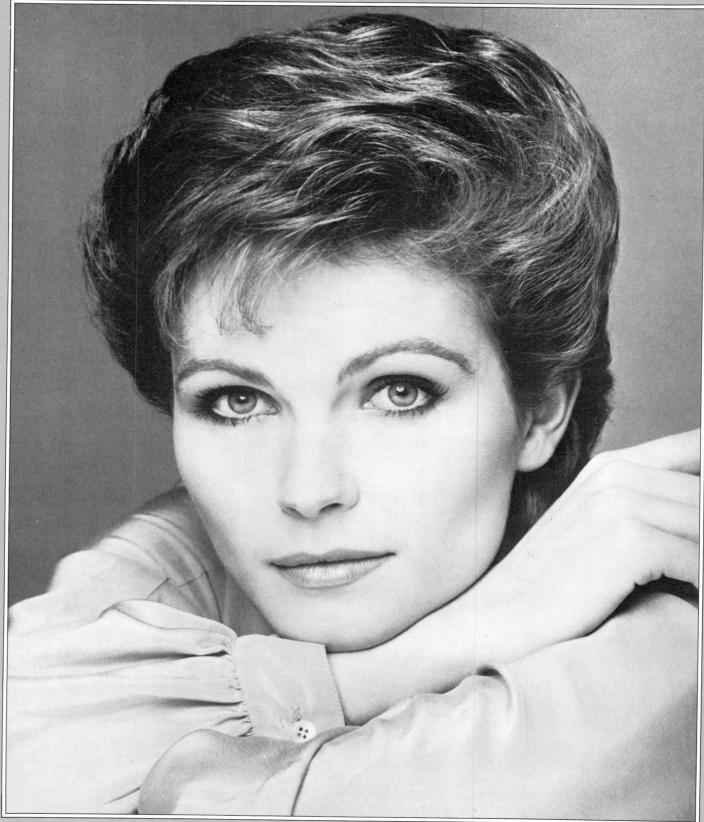

Introduction

Despite its title, *Hair Magic* is esentially a practical manual, full of ideas, information and advice covering every aspect of hair. It is a book not only for the fashion conscious few with money to spend and time on their hands but also very much for those who work, either in the home or in an office, and who cannot spend either time or money on elaborate hairstyles.

Chapter I, 'The Miracle of Hair' considers the myths and legends associated with hair that have been passed down through many generations. A brief history of hair styling through the ages is included, from Saxon times through to the present day.

Chapter 2, entitled 'Healthy Hair' looks at how hair is affected by your state of health and how the condition of your hair is not only indicative of your lifestyle but also, surprisingly, an accurate barometer of your mood. The chapter sets out how hair changes through the different stages of the life of an individual – from the delicate and finely-textured hair of a baby, through the full-bodied locks of a young man or woman, to the rather more delicate, and possibly balding, head of hair of an elderly person. It also discusses the onset of and reason for 'greying' hair and the resultant changes in texture, and contains a chart which lists the different types of hair and itemizes points which will help you to recognize your hair type.

There is advice on how to handle your hair on holiday, particularly in the summer months when you may well be on the beach and the authors explain in depth the effects of different climates and environments. For example, different hair treatments are required for those who live in towns or cities to those who live in the country. The harmful effects of alcohol and smoking are also covered and the importance of maintaining a proper diet, especially when pregnant, and of taking regular exercise, is stressed.

In the third chapter, 'Washing You Hair', the authors discuss the various types of shampoo and say which will suit different types of hair. There are detailed instructions for washing and shampooing both adult and children's hair, plus an analysis of many hair and scalp conditioners available on the market and how to use them to their fullest advantage.

Chapter 4, 'Drying and Styling' outlines the three basic methods of drying and styling your hair after it has been washed and shampooed. The chapter explains how to use pin-curls and ordinary rollers as well as electrical styling appliances such as heated rollers, curling tongs (curling irons) or hot brushes and there is a full account of the various types of hair dryers – both hand-held and hooded varieties.

The text also outlines the use of mousses, gels and hairsprays to hold the styled hair in place as well as the use of 'instant colours' and emergency rescue operations necessary for special occasions when your hair is limp or tired.

'Cuts and Cutting' is the title of Chapter 5 and it considers the many factors which should be taken into account when choosing a cut. The advantages and disadvantages of both the bob and the layer cut are discussed and step-by-step illustrations show how to achieve these cuts at home using the basic cutting tools and techniques employed by hairdressers.

There is a section on how to cut and trim different types of hair, including children's hair and another, equally important, section which deals with the care and trimming of beards and moustaches.

The chapter concludes by stressing the importance of finding the right hairdresser to care for your hair. He or she must not only be a good hairdresser but also someone who understands and appreciates your personality, lifestyle and, most important, how much money and time you are able to spend on the care of your hair.

Chapter 6, 'Colouring Your Hair' covers every aspect of this complex and exciting area of hair care and deals with temporary, semi-permanent and permanent colouring. There are sections on bleaching, using natural dyes, choosing colours to suit you, and how to achieve exciting special effects as well as highlighting and tipping. Checklists, charts and diagrams are included for rapid reference and to simplify, as far as possible, the complicated processes involved in techniques used to

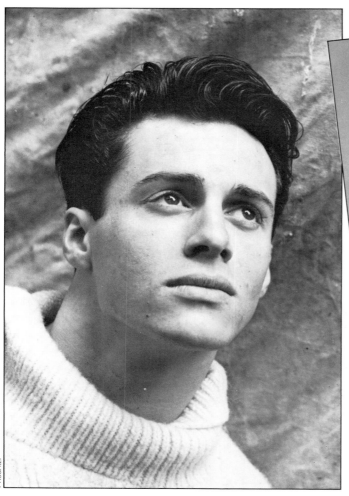

Phountzi

L'Oreal

colour hair.

The risks of colouring your hair are explained and it is emphasized that colouring or bleaching may have harmful effects on your hair unless great care is taken to make sure that the hair is revitalized and that the natural oils removed by the colouring or bleaching treatments are replaced with the use of the correct shampoos and conditioners.

Chapter 7, 'Waving and Straightening', outlines modern-day perming and relaxing or straightening techniques. There is a brief history of perming, together with an outline of new developments which show how permanent waves work and how to achieve them – both at the hairdressing salon and at home with do-it-yourself perming methods. The latest products and techniques for relaxing or straightening hair are discussed, together with a detailed account of how you can straighten your own hair.

The problems that can arise when waving or straighten-

ing your hair are clearly explained and the authors emphasize that it is vital to use whatever treatment you have bought on a small section of your hair first, before you begin the overall treatment, in order to check that the preparation is right for your hair. Again, the need for proper care and conditioning treatments is stressed.

Adapting hair to suit changes of mood and environment to achieve an overall look has become an important element of hair fashion today. Chapter 8, 'Dressing Up Hair' shows the versatility of hair and the various techniques which can be used to achieve magical changes and effects. Long, medium and short hair are all covered and there is a six-page step-by-step section devoted to a wide variety of styles suitable for all lengths of hair.

Accessories are essential features of the hairstyles of today and the latest hair 'add-ons' are set out in detail together with some exciting and innovative ideas for their use.

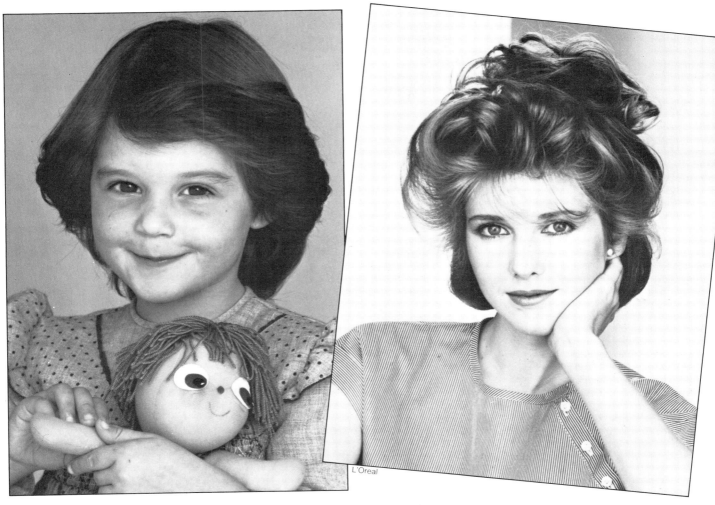

L'Oreal

Chapter 8 also outlines the uses of switches, hairpieces and fashion wigs. Party styles and hairstyles particularly suited to those people who have to wear glasses are shown, as well as some very special hairstyles to wear with hats.

Chapter 9, 'Thinning Hair and Hair Loss', caters for those suffering from thinning hair or baldness. Treatments, cuts and styling are covered in detail for those who no longer have an abundance of hair. Baldness in men, women and children is considered and there is a subsequent section on hairpieces and wigs used to cover bald pates.

Hair transplants are a fairly recent innovation and, because of rapidly improving techniques over recent years, have become an increasingly popular option for those who are already partly bald. The advantages and disadvantages of hair transplants are taken into account, together with the different methods used.

The 'Conculsion' summarizes the most important elements in *Hair Magic* and is intended to be an *aide memoire* for achieving the maximum benefit from the book.

There are three apendices. The first on recipes for hair care comprises 5 pages of imaginative do-it-yourself recipes, both old and new, for shampoos and conditioners for all types of hair.

The second appendix is a two-page spread of stencils to use or to adapt for exciting spray-on hair colour pattern designs, ideal show-stoppers for parties and discos.

The final appendix, comprising 4 pages, concludes the book with an A-Z of hair problems. This provides a quick reference to a wide variety of both common and unusual problems relating to the hair and scalp, how to cure them and prevent them from recurring.

There is something for everyone in *Hair Magic* which contains plenty of information, innovation and ideas. *Hair Magic* provides you with the wand; it only remains for you to weave the spell and make the magic.

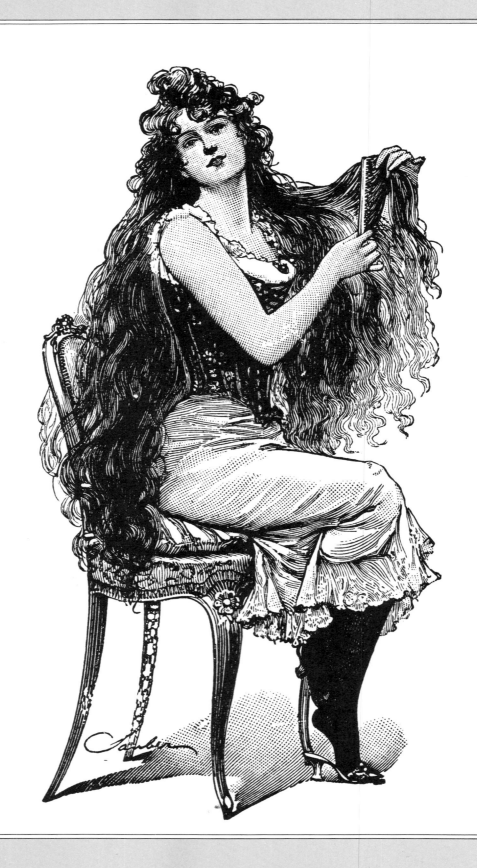

1
The miracle of hair

What does Samson have in common with fairy-tale princesses, Jean Harlow or nuns? Answer: an emotive association with hair. Hair identifies each of these people with a specific character trait, personality and lifestyle. Even though the qualities suggested – virility, virginity, sexuality and chastity respectively – are very diverse, hair is the common link that binds them.

Hair is the most revealing and important part of the human body in terms of social, sexual and psychological significance. It has been invested with mystical and magical powers, used to denote status and set fashion, and adapted as a means of attracting attention.

Fact and Fiction

There are many fallacies about hair, but some are stranger than fiction! Hair growth, for example, is thought to be related to sexual activity. A scientist, living celibate Mondays to Fridays on a remote island, noted that his beard grew more quickly during weekends when he resumed normal sexual relationships.

The morbid idea that hair continues to grow after death is probably a myth. Hair is an integral part of our living system and it is unlikely that hair growth continues after we die. Skin contracts after death and this makes it look as though the hair is still growing. Hair once removed from the head, however, can keep its colour for centuries.

Although you may not realize it, your hair can stand on end – just as it does with cats and dogs! The cause is the body's hormonal response which can make the small involuntary muscles – called the *arrectores pilorum* – contract. This gives us goose pimples and makes the root of the hair stand upright. Some soldiers from the World War 1 trenches were so affected by strain that their hair was said to have stood on end for months.

It is hard to imagine how hair can turn grey overnight, but such cases are reported quite frequently. If it happens, the causes are usually shock or a high degree of mental strain. The late Dr Agnes Savill, a dermatologist, cites several cases in her book *The Hair and Scalp*, including one in which a man was nearly blown up by

bombs twice in one night. His subsequent change of hair colour made him barely recognizable the following morning. Other cases reported tell of men whose hair and beards changed from black to white and back again three times in 30 years. The change from black to white was rapid, but the return to colour took five years.

Profuse hair growth is often seen as a symbol of virility in men. Samson's hair, the Bible tells us, held god-like powers. The ancient Greeks are known to have offered their hair in sacrifice to the gods. Scientifically, however, virility and a good crop of hair do not go together.

It is estimated that about one man in five starts to go bald soon after adolescence and is very bald by the age of 30. Another one in five retains a fairly full head of hair until after the age of 30, whereas the remaining three lose their hair more gradually.

Hair loss does not indicate a loss of sexual virility. On the contrary, baldness has been proved to be a result of an over-production of androgens, which are male hormones, essential for libido.

Hair development

No matter how different the outward appearance, all people's hair starts in the same way and at the same time: on the human embryo in the womb. All the hair follicles we will ever have in later life will be present below the skin over the whole body some three months before birth. These include the hair follicles for pubic hair and beards, which only become active at puberty.

As the body's hair growth patterns on the adult male and female are different, it is perhaps not surprising that hair has always played an important part in the sexual attraction between men and women. 'One lock of hair falling across the temples has an effect too alluring to be strictly decent', observed the painter William Hogarth in 1753. A thick, lustrous head of hair is not only a wonderful beauty asset, but its texture and quality can be sensuous in feel. The very fact that hair adds to our sex appeal has made hairdressing big business. Like a magician, the hairdresser can totally transform our looks.

Types of hair

Our hair, like our skin, depicts the physical characteristics of our racial differences. The texture and colour of hair vary widely between different races. Almost all Orientals have straight dark hair on their heads. Most Negroid races have tightly curled black hair. What are known as Caucasians, or the white races, can have anything from curly to straight hair that is usually, but not always, quite fine in texture.

Evolution has played an important part as the pattern of hair growth on head and body has clearly adapted to climate and life-styles. Races that have had to survive in strong sunlight have, over thousands of years, developed higher quantities of the pigment melanin in their skins. The melanin, which causes skin and hair to darken, protects against excessive ultraviolet radiation. As there is not so much sun in colder climates, there is less need for the protective melanin. As a result, inhabitants will have paler skins and hair that is brown or blond. Obviously, there are no hard and fast rules. Over the centuries, population migrations and the interbreeding of races have brought about an infinite variety of mixtures. Hair varies not only between different races but between individuals and hairs on the same head are not all the same texture or even the same colour. There is a sprinkling of red hair and fair hair on a reddish-fair person, whereas a brown-haired person will have hairs varying from red, fair and dark

among those of the predominant brown tint. The pigmentation cells of white hair contain air bubbles instead of the normal colouring matter. As a part of our ageing process, colour pigment fails to form and is replaced with air space, making the hair strand appear white or grey.

You can recognize your hair type by its texture, its appearance and the way it behaves. It is important to remember that different hair types require different treatment. For example, thin hair, which is usually soft and silky, does not have much bulk and therefore requires expert cutting to give it body and a style — helped by perming — combining curve and curl to give it volume. Thick hair, on the other hand, is heavy and may stick out in an unruly manner. It is often greasy at the roots and so requires conditioning. It also needs good cutting — club cutting (blunt cutting) is excellent for thick hair because it gives weight at the ends to hold the hair in place.

You can choose whatever you want in the way of a hairstyle, but if you want to look good it is important to remember your hair type when you decide what you want. There are only three basic hairstyles: short, medium and long. It is wise to think of keeping your hair short if you have curly and, particularly, coarse hair. Thick straight hair, however, can be worn long, while medium length hair suits most hair types.

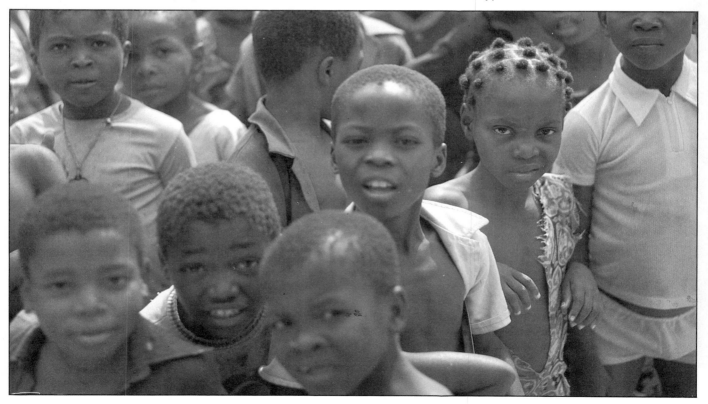

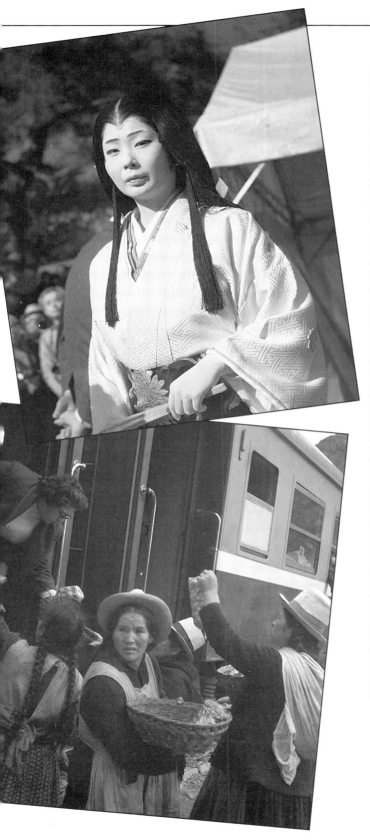

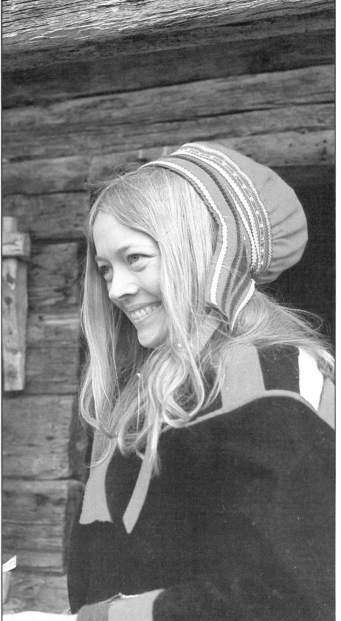

Far left: *These children, from the Central African Republic, have a typical Negroid hair type which is tightly curled and matt black in appearance.*

Top left: *Most Orientals have straight black hair which has a considerable gloss. This Japanese woman is wearing traditional dress and appropriate hairstyle.*

Above: *This Finnish girl has what most people regard as a typical Caucasian type of hair. Scandinavian hair is usually blond, straight and fine in texture.*

Left: *South American Indians are part of the Mongaloid racial group. Indian hair is straight and black, but less glossy than that of Orientals.*

Hair through history

Throughout history women have been plaiting, braiding or putting up their hair to create styles that are either practical or flamboyantly fashionable. In twelfth century England, as women emerged from the Saxon into the Norman period, they abandoned the head-covering veils to publicly display their hair. The fashion was to wear the hair parted in the centre with two plaits (braids) arranged to hang down in the front. The plaits were bound with ribbons and decorated with tassels or metal cylinders to give them the appearance of greater length.

Some centuries later in Louis XV's France, hair was being dressed up to most exaggerated heights, with lace and ribbons, pomades and animal fats and powderings of fine flour. During the reign of Louis XVI in the eighteenth century, his wife, Queen Marie Antoinette, is said to have worn headdresses so high that she had to kneel on the floor of her carriage to get to a ball as there was insufficient head room to accommodate her seated.

These excesses were brought to an abrupt end with the French Revolution and the terrors of the guillotine, when women aristocrats had their hair cut short at the nape of the neck before being beheaded. This short hair style was taken up by many women in France, especially if they had relatives who had been guillotined, and became known as the *à la victime* style.

By Victorian times, hair had grown long again and in the early nineteenth century was worn in chignon styles at the nape of the neck. By the middle of this century styles were dressed higher on the head, and by the beginning of the

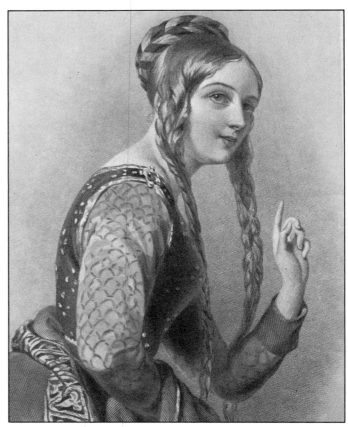

present century hair was again being dressed piled on top of the head.

During the First World War, a great many women were becoming part of the work force for the first time, and for practical reasons, hair was bobbed short. For the less emancipated woman who still preferred to keep her hair long, it was dressed in coiled 'earphone' braids – which was the last major braided style.

Throughout the ages, hair has been a symbol not only of sexuality, but of shame and chastity. The 'prison crop' in many gaols, when prisoners had their hair cropped short all over, is one example. Collaborators with the enemy in wartime were punished by having their heads shaved; the same treatment was meted out to witches. It was the custom for nuns to have their heads shaved as a symbol of chastity and unworldliness. In many cultures, women are required to put up their hair when they marry.

Above: *Eleanor of Aquitaine, King Henry II's wife, shown wearing hair in the style of the period, 1122-1204.*

Left: *An illustration of a French lady's head dress from the year 1771, showing the outrageous and exaggerated height and dressing which was fashionable at the time.*

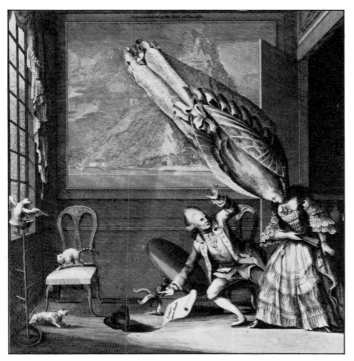

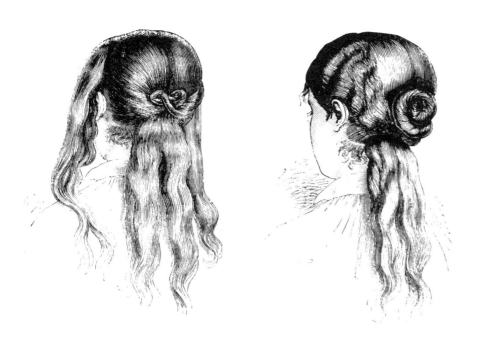

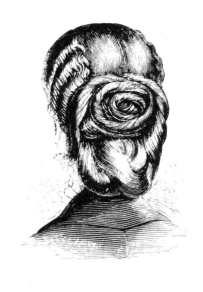

Above: *Three step-by-step illustrations from a ladies' magazine of the 1870s, showing a fashionable young lady's coiffure.*

Left: *The coiled braids of the 1920s resembled earphones.*

The wonder of hair

It is in the follicle that the birth, growth and death of the hair occurs. The hair follicle can be compared to a 'factory' with the actual manufacturing part, the papilla, as its bulb-like base. To think of the papilla as a 'root' is a misconception. Even when a hair is plucked out, the papilla stays behind and starts making a replacement hair. The papilla is rich in minute blood vessels. Connected to the hair follicle by a small duct is the sebaceous gland which supplies the natural oil or sebum to nourish the hair. Brittle or dry hair often suffers from a deficiency of sebum, whereas oily hair may result from an excess of it.

A hair lengthens only because a new piece of shaft is continually emerging from the papilla. This, in healthy people, occurs at a rate of about ½ inch (1.25 centimetres) a month, while in exceptionally fit people, it can grow as much as 7 or 9 inches (18 or 22 centimetres) a year. The hair shaft consists of three layers: the outer layer, also called the cuticle; the second layer, called the cortex; and the innermost layer, the medulla.

The cuticle is formed from tiny overlapping scales, similar to the scales of a fish or tiles on a roof. If you want to feel the roughness of the outer layer, draw your fingers through the hair from end to scalp. It will give you a sensation of 'going against the grain'. Like fingernails, the cuticle is transparent and does not affect the colour of the hair. When combed smooth, the hair looks soft and shiny, but when combed the wrong way, the hair can become dull and rough in texture. Improper handling of the hair and the use of harsh chemicals in dyes and shampoos can cause the layers of the cuticle to tear and loosen. When the hair is greasy, the cuticles tend to get clogged, giving a dull, lifeless appearance.

It is in the cortex, the second layer of the hair shaft, that the hair's natural colour matter, melanin, is found. The cortex comprises a great many long fibres which give the hair strength and suppleness. The fibres of the cortex separate readily and appear to be held together by the cuticle. Buried within the numerous fibres is the medulla, the innermost layer composed of spongy, cellular tissue. Within the medulla there are very few melanin-producing cells to provide colour. In very fine hair the medulla is often absent altogether.

The scalp covers an area of approximately 130 square inches (20 square centimetres) and the total number of hairs on it varies. The average human head has around 100,000 strands of hair. Blonds can have as many as 140,000, whereas redheads have fewer than usual only around 90,000 hairs on their head. Generally speaking, men's hair is coarser than women's. If we take a greatly magnified cross-section of an average straight hair, we see that it is round in form. Curly hair tends to be elliptical, whereas Negroid hair is kidney-shaped and nearly flat on one side. Orientals' hair, which is always straight and round in form, is well supplied with oil, whereas in contrast Blacks' hair tends to be dry. Blond hair tends to be fine

A CLOSE LOOK AT THE HAIR AND SCALP

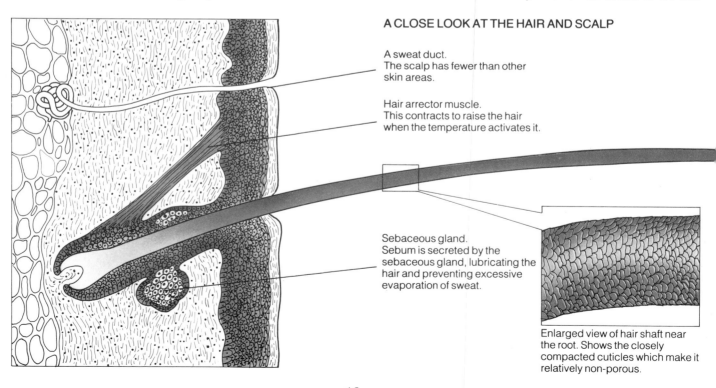

A sweat duct.
The scalp has fewer than other skin areas.

Hair arrector muscle.
This contracts to raise the hair when the temperature activates it.

Sebaceous gland.
Sebum is secreted by the sebaceous gland, lubricating the hair and preventing excessive evaporation of sweat.

Enlarged view of hair shaft near the root. Shows the closely compacted cuticles which make it relatively non-porous.

and curly hair coarser.

When the hair leaves the follicle, that is, when it actually shows on the surface of the scalp, it no longer receives nourishment from the papilla and, to all intents and purposes, it is dead. The hair remains in this state for about six years (some people believe it to be as long as 10 years), until it falls out and a new hair is produced in its place. Fortunately, the growth stages are staggered and even if something like 100 hairs a day are shed this is unnoticeable in the whole head of hair.

From a purely functional point of view, hair is an immensely valuable asset. It is present on almost all warm-blooded animals and its purpose is to prevent heat loss from the body and to maintain an even temperature on whatever part of the body the hair grows.

Eyelashes help to guard the eyes against flying dust and grit; the eyebrows act to channel perspiration away from the eyes; and the most luxuriant hair growth on humans – the hair on the head – also provides protection. Hair covers the skull against the burning rays of the sun and, to a limited extent, gives a protective cushion against glancing blows and the risk of scratches and abrasions.

Hair is a most durable substance and there are many instances of it having survived centuries without rotting, recorded when tombs have been opened and burial grounds disinterred. Perhaps one of the most noted examples of this is the mummified corpse in the British Museum's famous Egyptian Room. Dating back some

4,000 years, the body was dried and preserved by the warm desert sands where it had originally been buried. Still attached to the skull are several wisps of perfectly preserved hair.

Since earliest times, men and women seem to have known that hair can improve or detract from their looks. Length, colour, texture and cut have played an important part, not only in fashion, but in reflecting status and life styles throughout the centuries.

No other part of our body is as easily changed as our hair. If we do not like the shapes of our noses and chins we cannot cut them off and grow new ones. They cannot be altered except by plastic surgery. Hair, on the other hand, seems infinitely pliable. Cut it, and it will almost certainly grow again, and it can be set and shaped in very many different ways. At the same time, virtually every hairstyle we have today will have had its origins in previous eras. From the bleached hair of Roman women to the blue, orange and green dyes used by Anglo Saxons; from the short cuts in Tudor times to the long curls in the seventeenth century . . . some time, somewhere it has probably been done before.

Good hairdressers have the ability to make the most of our hair. For example, they can transform a nondescript grey mop into a radiant red head of hair. The imperfections on our face can be minimized and the attractive features emphasized. A good hair-do will not only make you look different; you will feel different as well.

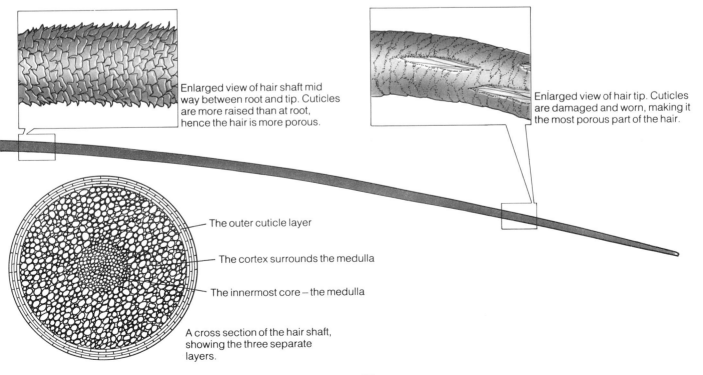

Enlarged view of hair shaft mid way between root and tip. Cuticles are more raised than at root, hence the hair is more porous.

Enlarged view of hair tip. Cuticles are damaged and worn, making it the most porous part of the hair.

— The outer cuticle layer

— The cortex surrounds the medulla

— The innermost core – the medulla

A cross section of the hair shaft, showing the three separate layers.

17

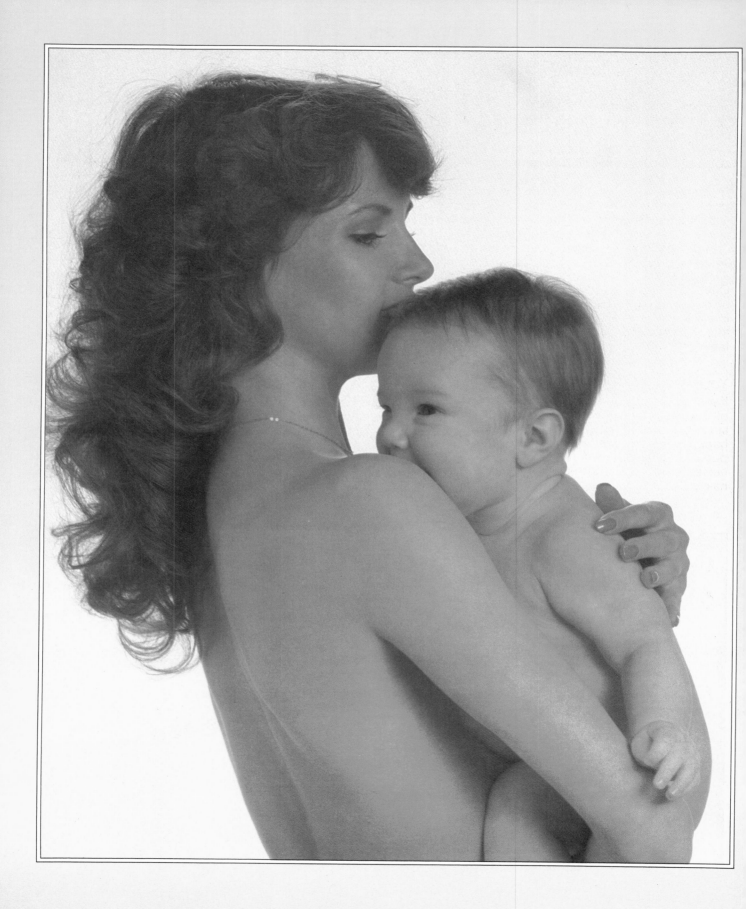

2
Healthy hair

One of the first parts of the body that will reflect your state of mind is your hair. Your hair and mental condition are so intertwined that an experienced hairdresser can guess by the condition of your hair whether you are depressed or feeling on top of the world.

Your mood and hair

If your hair doesn't look lively, chances are that you will not be feeling lively either. The reason is that stress can severely constrict the blood flow to the scalp. When this happens, hair growth is slowed down and the invisible papilla with its underlying system of blood vessels and nerves fails to receive the nourishment to produce healthy hair in the first place.

Although the effects will not be immediately noticeable, as it takes several days for healthy hair to react to the reduced levels of nourishment, once hair is starved of an efficient blood supply its healthy appearance will deteriorate dramatically. Within a few weeks it will be out of condition, limp, dull and lifeless. Unfortunately, it takes a long time for the hair to get back to its former healthy condition once a good state of health and proper nourishment have been re-established, but eventually its condition will respond to the improved blood supply and it will return to its former healthy look.

Many other factors affect hair growth, including your diet, the season of the year and even the time of day. Experiments have shown that hair grows faster in summer than in winter and that its growth is at its most rapid when exposed to sunlight. It seems that any type of light does, in fact, effect growth because the hair grows more slowly by night and faster during daylight hours, although, of course, this is not something we can detect for ourselves.

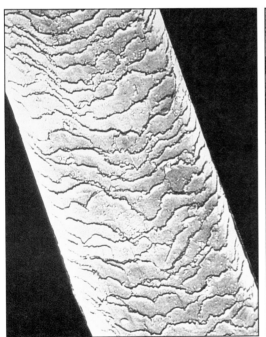 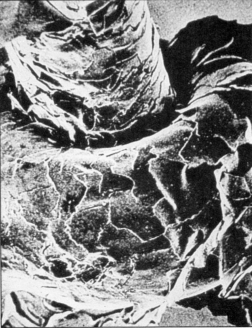

Far left: *Healthy hair which is in good condition has well compacted cuticles. This makes the hair appear glossy as the smooth surface reflects light. It also feels good and is less likely to tangle.*

Left: *Hair that is severely damaged shows a roughened and broken cuticle surface. The rough surface reflects little light and is liable to snag on its neighbours. This makes it look dull and liable to tangle.*

Age and hair type

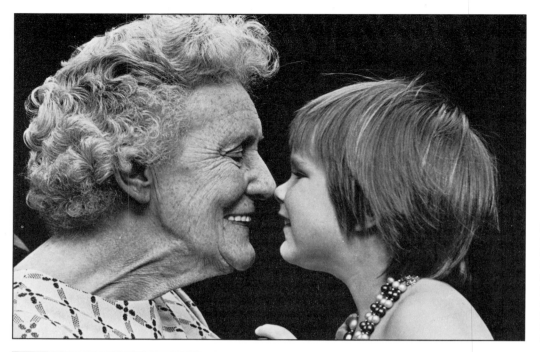

Left: *Hair changes its character as we grow older. This child's hair is thicker, more resilient, but less manageable than her grandmother's.*

Below left: *Hair can grow to an enormous length. Although not the longest on record, this Indian holy man has hair of prodigious length and bulk.*

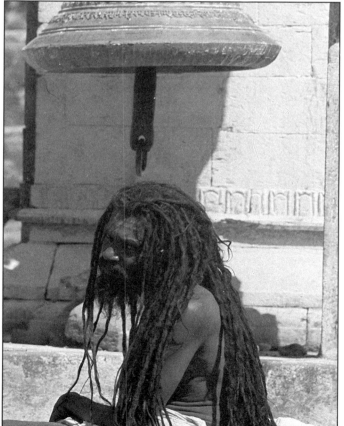

Our hair changes at different times throughout our lives, but why this should be the case is not completely understood. Before a baby reaches its first birthday, its soft, downy hair may already have changed colour, texture and curl. At the age of five or six, usually, when the first milk (baby) teeth are lost, the fine baby hair changes again and becomes more resilient. Often the hair is more difficult to comb and tangles quickly. Gradually, during puberty and into the teenage years, the hair becomes more manageable. Then it will more or less stay the same until it starts to go grey. When the hair is grey, it sometimes grows coarser but can also grow finer.

The average length to which a human hair will grow within its life-cycle if left uncut is from 22 to 28 inches (55-70 centimetres). In general, the lifespan of a woman's hair is a quarter longer than a man's. This could explain why women tend to produce longer hair. Hair that is more than 3 feet (90 centimetres) long is rare, but there are some notable exceptions. In the 1880s in America, Barnum and Bailey Circus gave star billing to the seven Sunderland Sisters who were reputed to have the longest hair in the world. Their thick, brown hair brushed the floor as they walked. Surprisingly, the all-time record is thought to belong to a man. In 1949, the *Toronto Morning Star* reported an Indian monk as having hair 26 feet long.

The rate of hair growth is fastest between the ages of 15 and 30 and is known to be slightly faster in women than in men. It does not grow at the same rate throughout its growth-cycle and this explains why hair can so quickly look uneven after it has been trimmed. Cutting hair of itself does not affect the growth rate. Although cutting the brittle ends will prevent hair from splitting and make the hair look full and healthy, it is impossible to alter the hair's growth pattern. As we age, the growth gradually slows down. Structural changes involving pigment, hair content and oil are all involved in the process that turns us grey. The pattern is fixed from the moment of conception, and the time at which pigment-forming cells stop transferring colour to the growing hair is governed by heredity.

The fact is that the hair we actually see sticking out from the scalp is no longer a living substance. It is made up of a protein material known as keratin which does not contain any living cells. So anything you apply to your hair once it has appeared cannot in reality affect its health or growth rate – even though it can make it look more shiny and beautiful – because it is actually dead.

The natural oils secreted by the oil glands attached to the follicles cannot reach far enough to lubricate the entire strand of hair. That is why the ends become starved as the hair shaft ages.

Hair type

There are many factors that go towards making up a good-looking head of hair, and the first factor to be considered is: what type of hair have you got? The answer to this question will govern how you have your hair cut, what type of style you wear, your shampoo and conditioning programme, and the setting techniques that give it its style.

It is important to recognize your hair type by its texture, its appearance and the way it behaves.

Thin hair is usually soft and silky but it does not have enough bulk to carry it through anything but the simplest of styles. This type of hair is more common a problem for the blond. It needs expert cutting to give the impression of bulk and a style that builds in volume with curve and curl. Perming is a great advantage and will give body to hair that otherwise might prove extremely difficult to handle.

Thick hair is heavy and grows in abundance all over the head, often sticking out rather than growing neatly downwards. It is often greasy at the roots, where the oil collects, and dry at the ends, so it needs plenty of conditioning treatments. It also needs good cutting to control the shape and benefits from club cutting (blunt cutting) to give weight at the ends to hold the hair in place.

Fine hair is thin in texture but quite often there is a lot of it, so it does not lack for volume and bulk but is generally fly-away and difficult to control. It does not hold a set well and is difficult to perm, so it looks its best cut in a short style or chin length at the very longest and layer cut

(layered) for graduated shape. It is important not to confuse thin hair with fine hair.

Coarse hair often feels harsh to the touch and lacks elasticity, which means it has to be handled with extreme care. It usually holds a style well, and so responds to roller setting. It needs to be club cut (blunt cut) for best effect if worn straight. This type of hair is difficult to keep shiny, so it benefits from regular conditioning. There is a tendency towards premature greyness so there is often a need to camouflage with colour at the onset of greying.

Curly hair is one of the strongest kinds of hair because it has lots of natural elasticity. It needs to be controlled through large roller setting techniques, by 'ironing' out with curling tongs and even by perming – to substitute larger curls for small frizzy ones. Layer cutting (layering) techniques can help to tame the frizz and hairspray is an important aid against damp weather.

Straight hair is difficult to manage. It does not maintain a set for very long, can look limp very quickly and looks really unattractive if allowed to get greasy. It is at its best with a really superb haircut such as a mid-length bob that makes the most of the straight lines and plenty of conditioning to make it glossy. A perm can make it frizz.

Hair style

Having taken your hair type into consideration, decide what length you like to wear your hair and choose the style most suitable for it.

Short hair is practical and easy to manage. It suits the 'petite' style of figure and is especially good for hair that is naturally curly and hair that is coarse. Regular cutting is essential to keep the line neat. A short style is useful if you have to let your hair get out of condition and need to cut off split ends and porous tips.

Medium length hair can be worn by most hair types. It suits a round face and helps balance a pear shaped face that is slim at the forehead, but full at the jawline. It is good if you like to try new accessories or different styling techniques. Medium length hair can be club cut (blunt cut) into straight bobs or layered to control unruly curls.

Long Hair is very suitable for thick hair that is well cut. It suits coarse hair that sets easily and it may be possible to have a leonine mane of curls that is flattering for strong features. However, avoid long styles if you have a particularly long face. Make sure to maintain long hair in the best possible condition – damaged hair tips tend to split and give a frizzy fish-hook effect that is unflattering.

Your hair on holiday

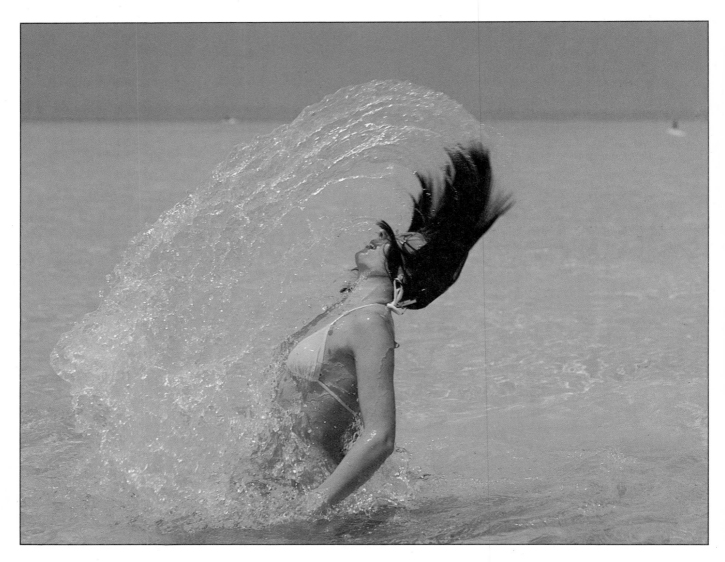

Whether your hair is oily or dry can be greatly influenced by climate. This is one thing to bear in mind when you go off on holiday. Forewarned is forearmed and the better prepared you are for a change in environment, the fewer problems you are likely to have. Do you know, for example, if the water is hard or soft? This may not sound important, but it could have a bearing on the type of conditioner you should take along. In very cold climates, when there is low humidity, hair becomes fly-away because of a high level of static electricity, and if you want it to behave, you may need a heavy conditioner. In a soft, temperate climate, a gentle shampoo and very light conditioner will be ideal. On a sight-seeing city holiday, where the atmosphere is dirty, your hair will reflect it unless it is shampooed often.

When you are on holiday, the need to relax applies to your hair too. This is when an easy-care style – one that doesn't need constant attention with careful setting – will really be a winner. From the minute you set off, the odds are somewhat stacked against your hair. Pressurized cabins in aeroplanes have a very low humidity and therefore tend to dry out the hair. After months of eating carefully, you are now tempted to go on a binge, often with less than healthy hotel meals . . . and a fair share of cheap alcoholic drinks. Along with drinks, you'll be spending many a happy evening in smoke-filled bars. As hair is porous, unless you take care it will look and smell nasty.

One good thing, though, is that you'll probably have plenty of time on your hands, so you can take the extra care which is essential, whether you go on to the beach or have a couple of weeks skiing in the mountains. It is best to start your preparations well in advance, so that by the

22

time you leave, your hair is in good shape. If you are planning a change of style, don't leave your hairdressing appointment too late, much better to have it done a couple of weeks before departure, having it trimmed the day before if necessary, so that you can really get used to it first. Don't risk going to a local hairdresser during your holidays, unless he or she comes highly recommended.

On either winter or summer holidays, you will need to protect yourself from the ultra-violet rays of the sun, which not only bleaches the hair but makes it more porous and liable to damage. At the seaside, the bad effects are made worse by the combination of ozone and salt water. To compensate for the extremely harsh, drying effects, give your hair an extra treat by applying a conditioning treatment while you're suntanning on the beach. After rinsing it when you've had a swim – which is just as important with chlorinated swimming pools – simply comb the conditioner through, concentrating on the ends of the hair. Then cover with a scarf and leave until you get back to the hotel when you can give it a good shampoo.

Oily hair may improve in the open air, but sea water will make strands brittle and bright sunshine discolours hair particularly if it has been tinted or highlighted. Ultra-violet rays from the sun can also penetrate through clouds and even through water, so protect your hair at all times. If you cannot bear to wear a hat or scarf, the least you should do is apply a conditioner after rinsing, leaving it on until you get back to the villa or hotel.

One thing is an absolute must: if you go swimming without a cap, either in the sea or in chlorinated swimming pools, always rinse your hair in normal water afterwards. It is very important so that if there is no source of natural water nearby you should bring your own. Save a few plastic lemonade (soda) bottles for the purpose if necessary. Should you run out of conditioner, you can always use a suntan lotion as a substitute. It can protect the hair as well as the skin in an emergency.

Remember that the sun's rays are actually intensified by the snow, so your hair needs even more protection during winter holidays. Harsh cold weather can expose hair to temperature extremes. When it is dry and freezing, it picks up static electricity and becomes fly-away. In damp weather, it can be miserably limp and unmanageably curly. During the winter months it is essential to wash your hair often and use lots of conditioner. Wearing a hat or scarf protects hair and helps conserve body heat.

When you want to set your hair, avoid using heated rollers when it is still damp. Wet hair is elastic and easily damaged, so even if you're in a hurry, allow it to get very nearly dry first if you possibly can. If necessary, to speed up the process, you can finger dry the hair with a blow dryer first, but when you do, keep it on a low setting.

A dry shampoo can come in handy, but use it sparingly and preferably no more than a couple of times a week. Dry

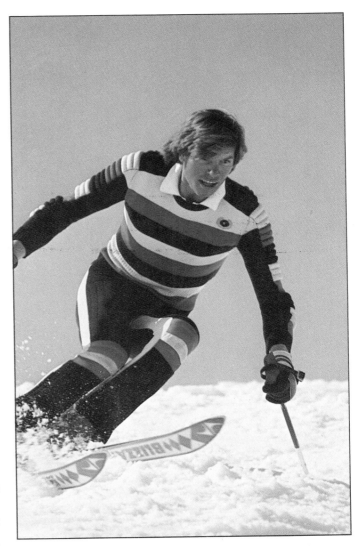

shampoos are based on talc or cornflour (cornstarch) which absorb oiliness from the hair and scalp and are then brushed out. However, if you use these too liberally, they can clog the pores and attract dirt.

A plait (braid) or ponytail can be convenient and cool for long or medium hair, but do take care not to apply too much traction. Elastic bands are out! Use those special, covered bands instead. Give the style a rest in the evening, and let it all hang loose and relaxed for a change.

If, in spite of these precautions, you still feel your hair has suffered as a result of your holiday, make an appointment with your hairdresser as soon as you get back. A deep conditioning treatment followed by a trim, which will get rid of any split ends, will help to put it back in shape.

Diet and exercise

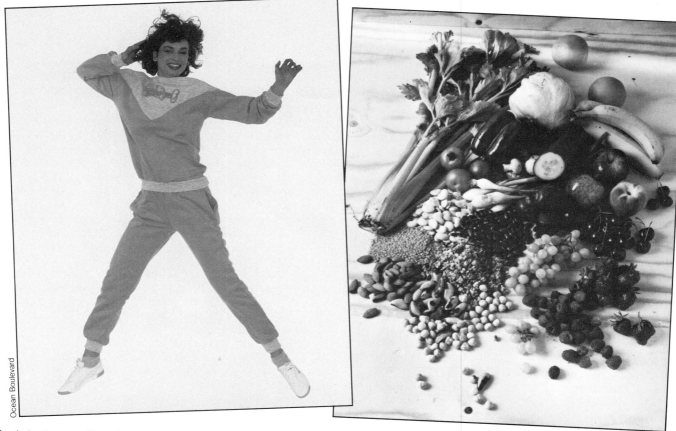

Ocean Boulevard

As it is the quality of the blood that supplies the papilla that will determine the quality of the hair, it is common sense to provide the hair, along with the rest of the body, with the proper nutrients. The more steps you can take to improve your overall health, the better the condition of your hair will be. The well-being of your entire body depends to a large extent on the substances you eat. It is believed that many ailments, from arthritis to migraine, can be treated and cured with a change of diet. Those who follow a strict diet may experience excessive hair loss two or three months after starting the regime.

Nutrition

Our hair is 97 per cent protein, which clearly indicates the importance of protein as part of our food intake. Protein cannot be stored by the body and must be replenished daily. It is most prevalent in meat, chicken, fish, cheese and eggs, but also plentiful in nuts, seeds, raw grains and beans. In fact, plant sources contribute 70 per cent of the world's protein supply.

Compared with the intake of proteins, fats and carbohydrates, the intake of vitamins is minute. Yet a deficiency in even one vitamin can affect and endanger the functioning of the whole body. There are two different types of vitamin: water soluble and fat soluble. The water-soluble vitamins such as the B-complex and Vitamin C are not stored in the body. This means that any excess of these vitamins is simply eliminated by the body, so you need to replenish them through food or supplements.

The fat-soluble vitamins, which include A,D, E and K, are stored in the body and, because of this, an excess of these vitamins can be toxic. Individual make-up, age, climate, sex and your general state of health are just some factors that indicate the amount and variety of vitamins a person needs. You may need advice from a doctor or dietitian before embarking on a vitamin programme.

The body can manufacture some vitamins for itself, but it is completely dependent on outside sources — that is food, drink and air — to provide minerals. Over 20 different minerals are now known to be essential in a healthy diet. One snippet of hair can tell the story of the complete mineral balance of the body. A few strands can act as a recording filament that reflects a deficiency in essential minerals and also an excess of toxic minerals such as lead.

The main role of minerals is to act as part of enzymes,

the protein substances needed to trigger off many bodily processes. The most abundant mineral in the body is calcium. With 99 per cent found in the bones, where it forms the basis of our skeleton and teeth, calcium is known to be an essential element for the rebuilding of bones. The remaining 1 per cent of calcium found in the blood has the important function of controlling muscle contraction and blood clotting. It can be important for hair because calcium determines the strength of our nerve reactions to stimuli. Emotional stress is thought to increase the amount of calcium lost by the body.

Iron was the first mineral to be widely prescribed by doctors, as long ago as 1831. Doctors realized that iron deficiency could cause anaemia and that women, particularly in their childbearing years, were most at risk. Anaemic blood does not carry enough oxygen and is frequently blamed for hair loss. Generally, the body is rather inefficient at absorbing iron from foods and it is known to be more readily absorbed from meat and fish than from vegetable products. For vegetarians, soy beans, yeast extract and almonds are the best sources and Vitamin C is known to help the body absorb iron.

More than 80 body enzymes — the substances that help chemical reactions take place in the body — are dependent on zinc as a co-factor to enable them to function correctly. Zinc is a crucial element in the proper development of skin, bone and hair and is known to be important in healing wounds. Research has shown that zinc deficiency can cause hair damage in animals and it could therefore do the same in people. Hormones in birth control pills are known to reduce zinc levels in the body and the mineral is also thought to be particularly important during pregnancy when deficiency could lead to abnormalities in the foetus. Seafood and meat are the richest sources of zinc, while whole grains, nuts, peas and beans are also important.

Eating

In our Western diet, fats generally comprise over 40 per cent of the total calory intake. A diet that incorporates a lot of fatty foods is not only bad for health but can often result in limp and oily hair.

A balanced eating plan means saying goodbye to junk foods that often contain harmful chemicals and a lot of salt. Salt can cause water retention and this, in turn, can deprive tissues of oxygen and lead to circulation problems.

For better health and hair, start at least one meal a day with a large salad, containing the greatest variety of greens and vegetables you can find. Gradually introduce more raw fruit and vegetables into your eating plan, substituting the occasional cup of tea or coffee with a glass of mineral water. The less food is processed, the

better. Two British researchers, Denis Burkett and Hugh Trowell, have helped to make us aware of the importance of fibre in maintaining health. Fresh fruits, leafy green vegetables, beans, nuts and wholewheat products are the kinds of food researchers say nature intended us to eat. Combined with exercise, a balanced diet comprised from a wide variety of foods is the best way to a healthy body and, of course, healthy hair.

Exercise

A healthy body needs a lot of exercise. Too little exercise can lead to poor blood circulation and this in turn can prevent sufficient oxygen reaching the tissues. When this happens, cell growth is slowed down because, without the oxygen, the body is unable to break down the nutrients in foods needed for energy and to nourish cells. Oxygen is also necessary to help our blood vessels remove carbon dioxide and wastes from the body through the lungs. In many people, particularly women, this elimination process is not as efficient as it should be. By far the most common cause is poor breathing. Deep, regular breathing should, therefore, be part of every exercise programme.

Although we are probably taller and healthier than our grandparents, our ancestors are likely to have taken far more exercise every day than we do. As we have cars and sedentary life-styles we now have to make time for exercise. The benefits are enormous: it not only helps to keep the circulation going, but also reduces stress and tension.

Just as you don't have to be a crank to be aware of the importance of your diet, nor do you have to become fanatical when it comes to exercise. 'Slowly does it' is the best way for most people. If you are unused to physical exercise, start off with some gentle stretching movements first thing in the morning and aim to take a brisk walk for 10 minutes each day. Slowly increase the amount of exercise and walking according to the time you have available. Don't overdo things, and exhaust yourself with too much sudden activity which may well give you aches and pains all over. If you are feeling uncomfortable, take heed! Your body is trying to tell you something and, if you take note, all will be well.

Posture

Bad posture, too, can have an adverse effect on the hair. By putting your back out of alignment, you can create tension in the shoulders and neck. Bad posture is one of the commonest effects of tension headaches. The muscles of the neck are strained and sore, because they have to support the weight of the head in an unnatural and difficult position.

One way of improving posture is with the Alexander technique. Invented by an actor, Frederick Matthias Alexander, this technique retrains people to adopt the correct posture by teaching them to be consciously aware of their body alignment in activities normally taken for granted, such as walking, standing or sitting.

Other techniques help improve body alignment, including yoga. Yoga works on the principle that if you take care of the mind, the body will take care of itself. In other words, the practice of yoga will help body and mind to integrate (the meaning of the Sanskrit word *yoga* is 'union'). Yoga combines exercise and meditation. It also concentrates on breathing as an important part of mind and body control.

The advantage of yoga is that it is not a strenuous form of exercise. A yoga-type shoulder or head stand will bring the blood supply to the scalp and help nourish the follicles. If you spend much of the day sitting behind a desk, try this head roll exercise for relaxation: close your eyes. Slowly bend your head forward and let your chin rest on your chest. Hold for a count of five and then very slowly roll and twist your head as far as it will go the left. Hold on again for a count of five, then roll the head back as far as possible. Hold for five and feel your chin and neck fully stretched back. Now move the head to the extreme right and hold again, before returning to the chin-on-chest position. Do this exercise at least three times, preferably more if you are prone to neck tension.

Yoga exercise is thought to stimulate the thyroid gland which is vital for healthy growth of hair and skin. Try to do it for at least 15 minutes a day. You owe it to yourself . . . and to your hair.

HEAD ROLL EXERCISE

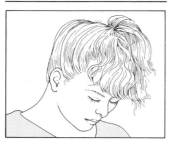

Close eyes. Bend head forward. Hold for a count of five.

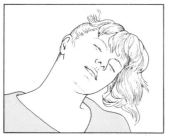

Roll head to the left. Do not exert force. Hold for a count of five.

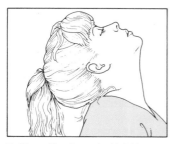

Roll head backwards. Hold for a count of five. Roll to right. Repeat.

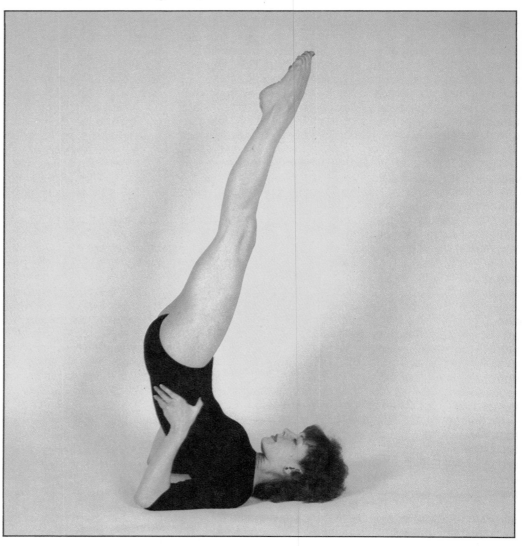

Pregnancy

Millions of cells make up the human body and each cell is a complex mechanism that requires fuel in order to live. Food and water provide the fuel and the means by which this fuel is converted into energy is called metabolism. The metabolism of one person is different from the next and it is the metabolic rate – the speed at which the body converts fuel into energy – that determines whether you put on weight quickly or whether, like some people, you can eat huge quantities without getting fat.

It cannot be stressed too often that anything that is harmful to health is going to be bad for hair and, the more you can do to stay healthy, the better the condition of your hair will be. Pregnancy is a time when you should take particular care. During pregnancy, one single cell will grow into a baby that contains more than six million cells – the fastest growth rate of any stage in human life. Most women go through pregnancy without problems, but even so, it is an enormous upheaval to the body causing wide-ranging hormonal changes in the process. The very least you should do is to watch your diet. This does *not* mean eating for two, but does mean ensuring an adequate intake of proteins, vitamins and minerals.

Protein is part of the structure of each of the cells of our body. It is needed to replace old tissues and to build new tissues. Proteins provide the chemicals that aid growth in childhood and help to repair or replace tissues and blood in people of all ages.

When pregnant you may have a vitamin deficiency without realizing it. For example, Vitamin B2 is not stored by the body and must be replaced regularly, especially during pregnancy and when you are breast-feeding. You are also likely to need more of this vitamin when you are taking the pill or if you suffer from symptoms of stress. In other words, it will help you 'keep your hair on'.

Often the hormonal effects of pregnancy are extremely beneficial. There are many cases when the rising oestrogen levels in the bloodstream reduce hair loss and leave both skin and hair glowing with health. This is because the placenta that feeds the growing foetus produces high amounts of female hormones. Unfortunately, once the baby is born and the placenta is expelled, the factory that has produced the extra hormones has gone. As the hormone levels are suddenly reduced, the body sometimes undergoes a shock and this can often cause the hair to fall out.

Normal hair loss is about 700 hairs per week but, two or three months after the baby is born, up to 30,000 hairs can be lost within a couple of weeks. Sometimes, this hair loss is delayed when the mother breastfeeds her baby. This is also due to the body producing the milk hormone prolactin.

During and just after pregnancy, you would be wise to avoid anything that will weaken your hair. By all means, have the hair trimmed regularly, but don't have it permed,

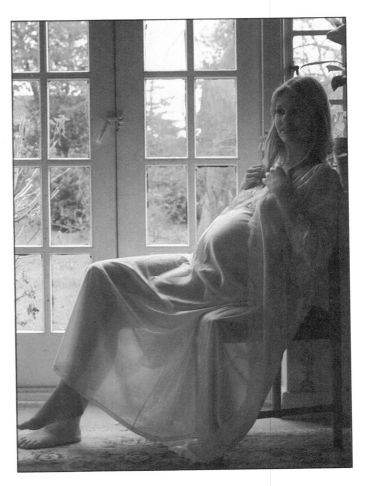

straightened or coloured for a while. Hair that grows during pregnancy is weaker and more sensitive than normal and this can present problems with perming and colouring. Avoid harsh drying methods, too. Do away with heated rollers and hot-temperature blow dryers and allow the hair to dry naturally

There is no denying that the extra weight put on during pregnancy places an extra strain on the body, so make sure you don't burden it further by putting on unnecessary pounds through careless over-eating and lack of exercise. In the last months, it is only too easy to convince yourself that your appearance doesn't matter and will soon get back to normal after the birth. So you let yourself go to seed. This is not only bad for your health, it is also bad for your morale! Pull yourself together and continue to do all the household chores and gardening as usual for as long as you can. By all means go out and enjoy yourself, and put your feet up during the day when you're feeling the strain. The right amount of work, rest and play will help keep your spirits up and more than ever, the better you feel, the more beautiful you and your hair will be.

Harmful factors

The effects of drugs can be detrimental to hair. If you are ill and are prescribed drugs such as cortisone or antibiotics, you may have to become philosophical and accept that the medicine is the lesser of two evils. If your hair starts to look out of condition or if hair loss occurs, you can probably be sure that the problems are only temporary. As soon as you finish the course, the hair will soon be back to normal. It is a good idea to tell your hairdresser that you are undergoing a course of drugs, as it may affect the way a perm or tinting treatment should be applied.

After a very severe illness, especially when there has been a high fever, hair loss can be profuse. When your health alters for the better, the hair will usually return and often all that is required is an adequate diet, lots of relaxation and fresh air with a fair amount of exercise.

As the condition of hair is totally dependent on the rest of the body, never take medication unless you are advised that it is really necessary. If you can do without sleeping pills and have a glass of warm milk instead, so much the better. Even the contraceptive pill, with its effect on hormone levels, can result in thinning hair. Vitamin pills cannot and should not ever be used to replace an adequate, healthy diet.

Dirt and dust in the air, lack of relaxation, a stressful job – all these are obstacles to having healthy and beautiful hair. If we are to keep a healthy head of hair in the next century, we shall have to treat it with extreme care to compensate for our polluted environment. Our hair is extremely vulnerable and many of the hairdressing processes we use can have a damaging effect. Chemical and mechanical damage created by perming and dyeing will become ever more likely as we grow older and our hair is subjected to constant abuse. Even a harsh shampoo or over-vigorous brushing of fine hair can cause problems. Is it any wonder, therefore, that trichologists are becoming very busy? They are not only consulted about hair loss, but also about hair that has come to look limp and lifeless.

Alcohol

Cut down on alcohol. If this is too great a sacrifice, remember that hard liquor has seven or eight times as much alcohol per volume as wine. Although the occasional glass of wine may help you relax, drinking a lot of alcohol can have a very bad effect on your health. Alcohol depletes the body of both B and C vitamins, is harmful to vital organs like the liver, and can make you fat in the process.

Like white sugar, the calories alcoholic drinks provide are empty of vitamins, minerals and fibre. In the same way as caffeine – which is present in tea and chocolate as well as in coffee – alcohol is a drug.

If you are weight-watching, bear in mind that many mixers, such as tonic water or ginger ale, are full of empty calories.

Smoking

Smoking is known to deplete the body of Vitamin C. Each cigarette is thought to destroy some 25 milligrams of Vitamin C, so if you cannot cut out smoking, do compensate by taking a supplement. Remember that the carbon monoxide from inhaling cigarette smoke enters the blood and destroys oxygen in the red blood cells.

Few smokers would deny that smoking is bad for you. At the very least, a hardened smoker must, however reluctantly, come to the conclusion that it is a dirty habit, objectionable and anti-social in any environment shared with non-smokers. The reason why so many people are still hooked is simply because it is so difficult to stop. Nevertheless, millions of people have done so and, almost without exception, have felt a great deal better for it. Go and see your doctor for advice.

Today, smoking is no longer glamorized. In Hollywood's heyday, in the 1930s and 1940s, film stars such as Bette Davis were never seen without their elegant cigarette holder. Today, on the contrary, one TV anti-smoking advertising campaign, aimed at young people stresses that smoking 'makes you smell'. A couple of young men look at an attractive girl in the same room and one dismisses her, saying to his friend: 'her hair smells; her breath smells; it is like kissing an old ash tray'.

This particular campaign never even mentions the harmful physical side effects that are thought to be smoking-related, such as the high incidence of heart disease, bronchitis and lung cancer. When you smoke a cigarette, after a few minutes, it causes the air tubes in the lungs to shrink and this affects your ability to breath efficiently. As it is the quality of the blood cells and the amount of oxygen in the blood that largely determines hair health, it stands to reason that smoking is going to be harmful both to hair and skin in the long term. Few heavy smokers can boast of a fine complexion or glossy hair.

It is simple enough to wash your hair to get rid of the smell, but less simple to improve your lungs' ability to breathe properly.

Pollution

We hear a lot these days about environmental issues and the problems connected with them that effect our daily lives. A major factor is pollution and the effect it can have on our health. Tests have shown that plants growing in fields or gardens alongside busy motorways, contain unacceptable levels of lead content. Anyone living in a major city knows that the air is fouled by exhaust fumes –

the evidence is visible enough in the form of smog or layers of dirt that accumulate quickly on any flat surface.

It needs no stretch of the imagination to realize that it is unavoidable that we are taking in similar layers of dust and dirt into our lungs and there is the possibility of toxins accumulating or spreading through our bodies. So pollution can have a detrimental effect from both within and without.

It is a problem that is being recognized in the industrial countries throughout the world and, gradually, moves are being made to control and cut down on the risks of urban pollution caused by motor car exhaust fumes, factory chimneys, etc. So, it is to be hoped that the dangers will be reduced in the future.

Meantime, there is no doubt that city living does take its toll on the condition of our skin and hair. Dust and dirt in the air leave a fine, dulling film clinging to the hair, especially if it is greasy. The city dwellers must brush their hair daily to get rid of the surface dust and shampoo much more frequently than others living in comparatively cleaner rural areas. Since over-frequent shampooing can rob the hair of its natural, protective oils, it is important to use a mild shampoo and regularly apply conditioning treatments.

There are other aspects of modern-day living that have a detrimental effect on the hair. One of the most common factors is the ever-increasing use of central heating. Where once we relied on fires – open, gas or electric – to provide a room with a focal heating point, we now tend to have our buildings heated throughout to the same overall temperature, which creates an artificially dry, hot temperature with reduced humidity. This can result in excessive moisture loss from the skin and scalp. With dehydrated skin there may be wrinkling and premature ageing or a peeling and flaky complexion. Excessive moisture loss can also lead to brittle fly-away hair through a build-up of static electricity that robs the hair of its elasticity, strength and shine.

If this happens you will need to replace the lost moisture with regular conditioning treatments such as hot oil applications, moisturizing or protein packs, to restore the hair to good condition. It is better still if, in the first place, you are able to prevent this loss of humidity from the air with the use of special humidifying equipment to counteract the effects of central heating.

By being aware of the everyday environmental factors in your life that can cause problems to the hair's health, you can combat them with conditioning treatments.

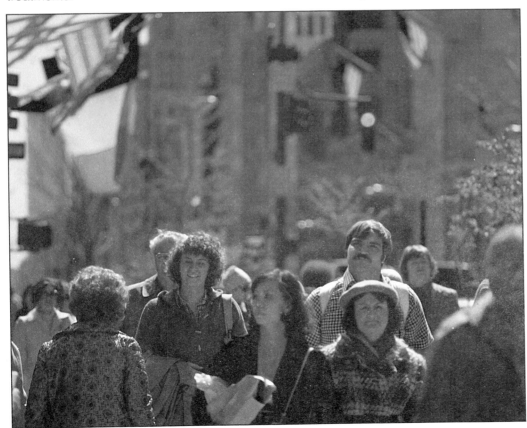

Every busy city, no matter how efficient its environmental controls, has pollution problems. Some cities are so badly affected they produce their own smog accumulation. Anything from dust and grime to carbon monoxide and lead can be found in the atmosphere. Industrial areas can be worse. Gaseous chemical waste is often released into the air and in combination with rain dilute acids and other harmful chemicals can be formed and spread over large areas and be carried for great distances.

Polluted environments present many problems for those who work in them and who want to retain healthy and attractive hair. The pollutants must not be allowed to accumulate, so regular hair washing is essential. To prevent damage by harmful chemicals it is also necessary to regularly condition hair. Perfumed and herbal rinses also help to remove that city smell which especially clings to greasy hair.

3
Washing your hair

To keep your hair in good condition you need to build up your own hair kit. What it contains will depend largely on your hair type and the style in which you wear it. This will dictate what kind of hairbrush you use, dryer, styler or rollers for setting, combs, pins and grips (clips), as well as the shampoos, conditioners and setting aids you choose.

A basic kit

A prime requisite is a hairbrush. Regular brushing keeps the hair free of dirt and dust and helps to bring out the hair's natural sheen. A wide-based brush with the bristles set in a rubber cushion is best for this. You will need a styling brush that has bristles set in a semi-radial (round) shape on a narrow base or a completely radial (round) brush to encourage curl and movement and for use when blow drying the hair. Ideally, the bristles should be pure animal hair – hog's or boar's bristle – but if a synthetic nylon bristle is used, be sure the ends are gently rounded and not sharp, as sharp ends could damage the hair.

You will need two or three combs. One with widely set apart teeth for use on wet hair, a (rat) tail comb, especially useful for picking out sections of hair when roller setting, and an ordinary styling and dressing-out comb with fine teeth at one end and slightly wider teeth at the other to cope with tangles. Natural materials such as horn and tortoiseshell are considered the best for the hair as they do not create static electricity, but there are good nylon and synthetic combs available that have been specially treated or coated to be anti-static. Make sure the teeth have a smooth finish and no ragged edges.

A selection of hair pins, clips and small combs will be necessary for sectioning off areas of the hair during home hairdressing sessions, and heated rollers, ordinary rollers, electric styling appliances, such as heated tongs, brushes and curling tongs, according to your hair setting requirements, are also needed.

A hair dryer is a basic piece of hair care equipment few people would be without and the one you choose will depend mainly on your hairstyle. It will most probably be a hand dryer (a hand-held blow dryer), although if you regularly roller-set your hair, a hood dryer is useful.

Again, depending on how you style your hair, you will have hairsprays and setting lotions. Sprays that come in aerosol form have attracted the criticism of environmentalists who maintain the gas used as a propellant escapes into the atmosphere and risks endangering the ozone layer that protects the earth from the more damaging of the sun's ultra-violet rays. Other preparations come in bottles with a pump action. Setting lotions are usually polymer-based liquids and come with a choice of colour to add the hint of a tint to the hair.

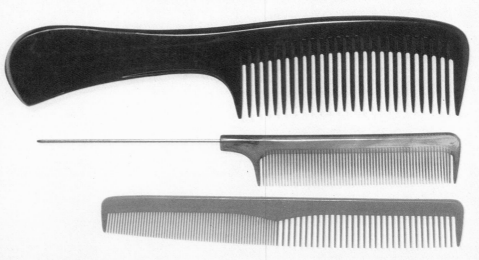

On the right is a selection of combs. The top one is ideal for wet hair because it is wide-toothed and therefore is gentle on the hair when it is in its most vulnerable state. The comb in the middle is a tail (rat tail) comb. The tail, which can be either plastic or metal, is used to section hair, for example when perming. The last comb in the selection is an all-purpose comb, perfect for holding the hair straight when cutting or trimming.

On the right the photograph shows one type of hand-held hairdryer and two alternative attachments, for brushing the hair whilst drying it. Below is a selection of brushes - left to right - two radial brushes, the first is usually used to create flip curls while drying the hair, and the second is ideal for creating larger curls or for curling a bob under or out at the ends. The third brush shown in the line up is a rubber cushion brush with plastic pins which does not pull on the hair because the rubber cushion 'gives' when the hair is brushed; the final brush, also rubber cushioned, has the same advantages, it can also give more volume to the hair and is ideal for the traditional '100 brush strokes'.

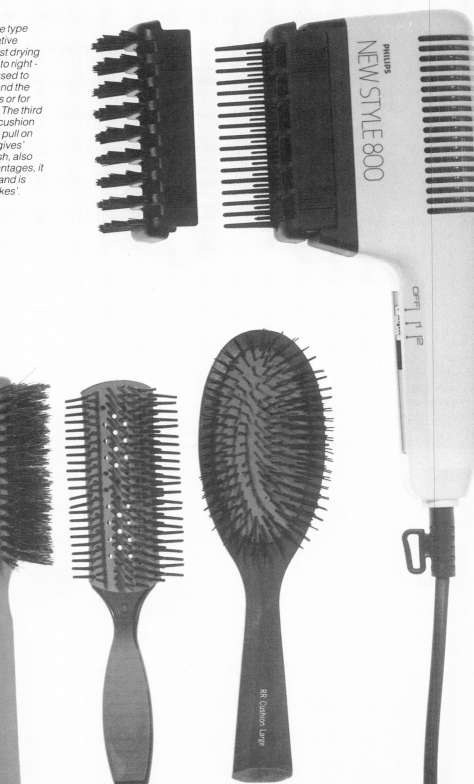

Shampoos

The average shampoo you buy contains around fifteen ingredients. It is made up of water, anionic and amphoteric surfactants – they provide the foaming and cleansing properties – a foam stabilizer to maintain a good lather, conditioning agents, a thickener to make the mixture easier to handle, fragrance, colouring, maybe a pearlizing agent to make the product look attractive in its bottle, and the particular ingredient that lends its name to the shampoo: lemon, jo-joba, rosemary, etc.

What very few of them actually contain is soap. Practically all shampoos made today rely on artificial detergents for their cleansing effect. There are basic reasons for the switch from soap that, until the beginning of the 1950s, was a basic shampoo ingredient. Soap is not compatible with hair or with hard water, because of its alkaline properties.

Hair, like skin, has a protective acid shield that acts as a natural guard against infection because germs and bacteria do not like an acid environment. This acid shield is described in the terms of a pH factor, which is a scale of measurement running from 1 to 14 to describe whether something is acid or alkaline. Taking the number 7 as neutral, then anything below 7 is acid and anything over 7 is alkaline.

The hair and skin have a pH factor of between 4.5 and 5.5, which make them both slightly acidic. It is important to maintain this acidic state if the hair is to be at its most healthy and manageable. Soap and alkaline products – such as permanent wave lotions and bleaches – rob the hair of some of its acidic properties and this can be damaging. The alkali causes the hair to swell and the outer cuticles to lift up, leaving the inner core of the hair vulnerable to the comparatively harsh action of shampooing, brushing or combing. A product with a lower pH more akin to the hair's natural pH of around 5 causes a slight shrinking effect so the cuticles lie flat and protectively close around each hair.

Another reason why soap is not considered good for shampoos is that, when used with hard water, the alkali content combines with the calcium and other minerals in the water to form a very fine deposit or 'scum' that leaves a fine white film on the hair which is difficult to rinse out. Detergents do not have this disadvantage and are more economical to use.

Only a few of the many soapless detergents are suitable for shampoos, however. They have to be readily soluble in water and easily rinsed out of the hair; they must offer no risk of irritating the scalp; and they must leave the hair manageable. All these requirements are met by a group of detergents called lauryl sulphates, which are made from vegetable fats, such as olive oil, castor oil and coconut oil.

The amount of lather a shampoo provides has little to do with its cleansing properties. In fact a perfectly thorough job can be done with a shampoo that does not foam, but as we tend to equate the effectiveness of a shampoo with the lather it produces, so foaming agents and foam stabilizers are used by most shampoo manufacturers for the customers' benefit.

Conditioning agents are probably among the most important ingredients in a shampoo. Because, no matter how mild a detergent is used, to have a cleansing effect it has got to remove the dirt and along with it the oil that is clinging to the hair shaft. Hair that is greasy can benefit from having more oil taken away than can dry hair, which is one reason why shampoos come in 'dry', 'greasy' and 'normal' hair formulations. Shampoos for dry hair will contain more emollient and conditioning agents than shampoos for greasy hair. This is why it is well worth spending time choosing the shampoo that suits your particular hair type.

As a general rule, other ingredients are used in too small a quantity to have a particularly noticeable benefit. Medicating agents, such as coal tar and zinc pyriothine, have antiseptic properties useful in treating dandruff conditions; lemon additives have a fresh attractive smell and counteract greasiness; and camomile may contain a little of its natural lightening properties for fair hair.

Shampoos that are made to add colour to the hair, of course, do contain a fairly active staining ingredient that remains on the hair after rinsing but, generally speaking, the effectiveness of added ingredients on the look and health of the hair is minimal.

There are two things which you must look for on a shampoo label: that it is acid-balanced – either stated as such on the label or identified as being a pH balance of between 4.5 and 5.5 – and that it is formulated for your particular hair type.

Then it is a case of selecting the type of shampoo you personally prefer – whether a liquid, cream or gel – the fragrance you like and the price you can afford. Generally speaking, you get what you pay for, and a shampoo that is very cheap is likely to lack some of the better emollient and conditioning agents that benefit the general condition and manageability of the hair.

Conversely, buying a very expensive shampoo does not mean it is going to do a miraculously better job than a cheaper one. You will be paying for a number of things needed to 'sell' an expensive shampoo, such as smart packaging, costly advertising campaigns and pricey perfume ingredients, which have little to do with the shampoo's actual efficiency. So it is often better to stick to a product which is simply packaged and well-enough established not to require a lot of unnecessary promotion, and as a consequence is reasonably priced.

Finally it is a case of using a shampoo properly, with gentle and thorough techniques that leave the hair clean, healthy and tangle-free.

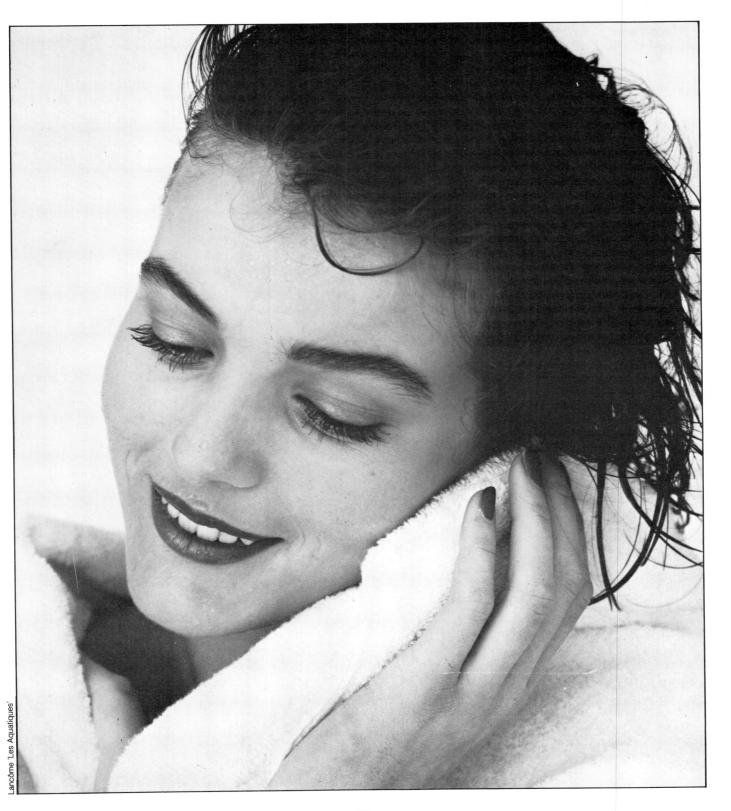

Adult hair

You need to shampoo your hair in order to remove dirt and oil from the scalp and leave the hair shafts clean and non-greasy. The scalp has oil and sweat glands, but because the scalp is covered with hair, grease and sweat tend to get trapped around pore openings and so it often seems more oily than the rest of the body.

How often you wash your hair depends not only on how greasy your scalp gets, but also on external factors as well. Pollution from a city environment, a hot climate, or the activities in which you indulge, such as an active sport or heavy physical labour that makes you sweat quite a bit, will affect the scalp. Fresh perspiration attracts dust and dirt and, when it dries, causes the scalp to itch.

Young women today wash their hair more frequently than their mothers did. For one thing there is a greater awareness of the importance of personal hygiene. Hairstyles are also more casual. Most people wear a wash-and-wear style rather than a formal dressing, so hair washing is far less of a chore than it once was.

On average, young people wash their hair two or three times a week, but greater frequency is not uncommon. Major hair care product manufacturers are catering for this trend with mild shampoos advertised for use every day.They are actively helping to promote a daily hair washing routine which can cause dry and out-of-condition hair if the shampoo chosen is too harsh.

How you wash your hair is quite as important as the choice of the right shampoo. You need to start by thoroughly brushing your hair to get rid of surface dust, dirt or hairspray and to ensure that the hair is tangle-free. Because hair is at its most fragile when wet, it can easily be damaged by pulling a brush against a stubborn tangle. Far better to eliminate that risk from the outset.

Having done so, wet hair thoroughly with water that feels comfortably warm to your scalp. Never have the water too hot – especially if your hair is greasy – as it can activate the oil glands and cut down the efficiency of the shampoo. For the same reason, when working shampoo into the hair or when rinsing do not use too vigorous an action as rough handling can also stimulate the oil glands.

If you wash your hair very frequently – say every other day – then one application of shampoo will be sufficient. For hair that is washed less frequently, however, if it is particularly greasy or extra dirty, two shampoo applications will be necessary. In such a case there will not be a lot of lather apparent with the first application, which will loosen the dirt and grease and soften the hair cuticle. Be sure to thoroughly rinse off the first application, which will take the worst of the grease and dirt away.

Then, you are ready for the main shampooing stage. Pour the shampoo into the palm of your hand, rather than tipping it on to the head as this can be wasteful if the shampoo is fairly liquid and runs into the basin (sink) instead of staying on the scalp. Spread the shampoo

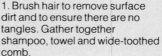

WASHING YOUR HAIR

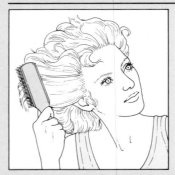
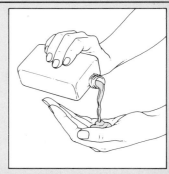

1. Brush hair to remove surface dirt and to ensure there are no tangles. Gather together shampoo, towel and wide-toothed comb.

2. Wet hair thoroughly with comfortably warm water and add shampoo, which has been tipped into the palm of the hand to the crown and front area of the head.

evenly through the hair from the front of the crown through to the ends, using a light circular massage motion.

Work the lather up to provide an effective cleansing of the scalp and through the lengths of the hair, taking care not to drag at the hair roots or pull on the hair. The cuticle will also be softened by the shampoo and will be in a raised state, so more inclined to 'catch' and tear or tangle.

When shampooing is complete you are ready to rinse, using plenty of warm running water. A shower or spray is best for rinsing, otherwise, emptying saucepans of water over your head will do until every trace of shampoo suds and residue is washed clear, the water runs crystal clear and the hair feels completely clean. One of the ways of finding out whether this stage has been reached is if the hair makes a 'squeaky' sound when rubbed between your fingertips – hence the origin of 'squeaky clean'.

Remember your grandmother always rinsing her hair with water that contained a few drops of vinegar? By all means, follow her footsteps, especially if you live in a hard-water area. Vinegar helps to give the hair a protective coating to form what is known as a 'liquid' shield that can also remove the dulling film often left on the hair by hard water.

Satisfied that all traces of the shampoo are gone, give the hair a final rinse with cold water to close the pores, gently squeeze excess water from the hair and wrap a towel around your head to blot the hair semi-dry. Do not rub, as that causes tangles, and do not use a brush, which is too aggressive for hair in a wet state. Instead, comb through gently with a wide-toothed comb.

Then set your hair in rollers or blow dry according to preference. If blow drying, a more glossy and smooth effect can be achieved if the hair is a little damper than for roller setting.

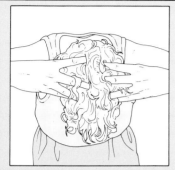

3. Rub shampoo through the hair to loosen dirt and grease and soften cuticle. If hair is particularly greasy, rinse thoroughly and apply more shampoo. Work into lather all over head.

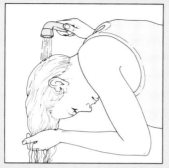

4. Rinse hair thoroughly with warm water from a spray, starting from the back of the neck, working water through hair, over scalp and down to the ends hanging over the basin.

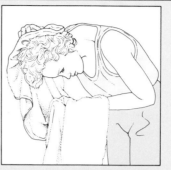

5. Stop rinsing when water runs clean and squeeze excess water from hair before blotting dry with a towel.

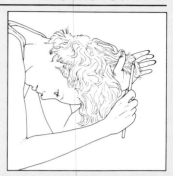

6. Use a wide-toothed comb to ensure hair is tangle-free, working from the ends upwards to scalp.

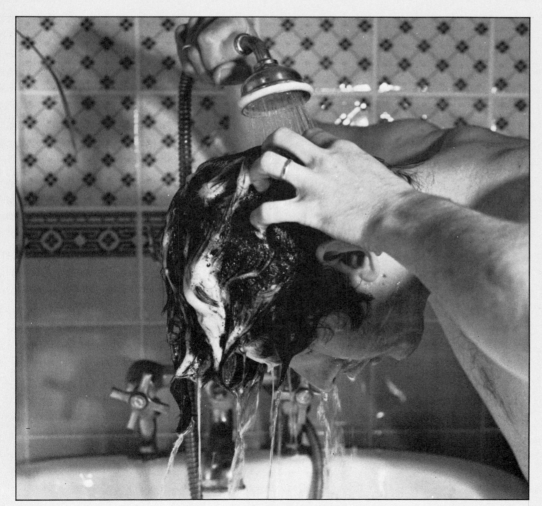

Men have always washed their hair more frequently than women, simply because, with the exception of a brief period in the late 1960s and early 1970s, they've usually worn their hair a lot shorter than women do. The daily shower makes it as easy to wash the hair as well as the face and body.

But daily washing, and especially with soap rather than a shampoo, can dry out the hair's natural oils and lead to a dry thatch rather than a head of shining, healthy hair. So it is quite as important for a man to take care in choosing the right kind of shampoo that is efficient enough to do a good cleansing job, yet mild enough not to rob the hair of its shine and lustre.

One lathering should be sufficient and the use of a conditioner should be regarded as a matter of course.

Children's hair

Mothers should make sure they have the right products and equipment to look after their baby's hair from the first downy fluff stage through to the thicker growth that starts coming through around the age of two years.

Even when your baby has very little hair, what there is needs to be kept scrupulously clean and it should be washed regularly, at least once a week. Baby shampoos are made with special mild ingredients that are gentle to the skin and do not sting the eyes. They are usually unperfumed to avoid any unnecessary risk of skin irritation and, because they are so mild, they do not need the special conditioning agents found in general shampoos. Other additives, such as foam boosters or thickeners, are also not considered necessary, and the shampoos are kept as pure and uncomplicated as possible.

In shampooing, what holds for the adult is true for the baby – not only must the hair be washed, but the scalp must also be thoroughly cleansed. Because a baby's head is so soft, mothers are often nervous of massaging enough to give a good shampoo. Firm but gentle massage should be used to work the shampoo into the scalp, but do not exert too much pressure because the baby's skull is still not totally formed and has a soft part – the fontanella – where the bony structure has not completely knitted over.

Rinse the hair well, holding the baby's head in a backward position and scooping water through the hair. You can avoid getting water or shampoo in the baby's eyes by using a shampoo shield. This is a halo-shaped frame with plastic attached, which clips around the forehead to block trickles of water running into the eyes.

The hair should be blotted carefully with a towel and then dried with gentle brushing. This should always be directed back from the forehead to the crown, and with upward strokes at the sides and back. This technique of brushing against the natural fall of the hair often helps to produce a soft wave or enhance the hair's natural curl.

A baby's delicate scalp requires a special brush and comb. The softness of the head and the fineness of the hair calls for an extra-soft bristle brush, which also needs to be treated with care and kept scrupulously clean. Similarly, a good-quality comb, made for baby-fine hair and with softly rounded teeth that will not scratch or

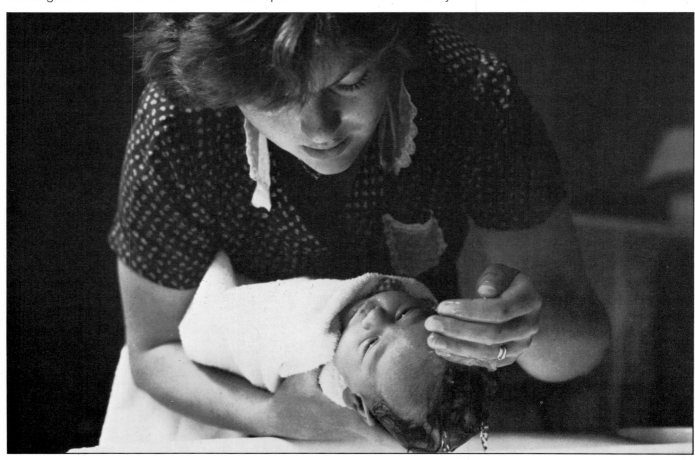

damage the scalp, should be used.

As your baby grows into a young child, the hair will gradually strengthen and the scalp will not be quite so sensitive, but care still needs to be taken over shampooing. A young child is far more likely to be aware of the unpleasantness of shampoo suds in the eyes. This will probably make him or her constantly reluctant to undergo the experience and can turn shampooing into a traumatic occasion for both parent and child.

The answer to this problem is to try to alleviate tensions and to deal with any unpleasantness as quickly as possible. Usually it is best to combine hair washing with bath time, then it does not matter how wet the child gets. Also it helps to prepare as much in advance as possible, so the actual shampooing is as straightforward as it can be. This will mean ensuring the child's hair is tangle-free before damping it down and that you have all the equipment and towels you need to hand so the job can be completed quickly and efficiently.

You will probably find the use of a shampoo shield helpful to stop water and shampoo suds running into the eyes or, alternatively, you can buy special goggles which protect the eyes and look a bit like a miniature piece of scuba diving equipment.

Make sure the water you use is not too hot and if you use a hand spray, be careful to hold it close to the head so the water will run through the hair rather than bounce off and spray the rest of the bathroom.

Leave the shampooing to the end of the bath time session, so that once you have finished with the final rinsing, you can take the child out of the bath immediately, wrap a warm bath towel around the child that is large enough to encompass body and head and allow the hair to be gently blotted dry.

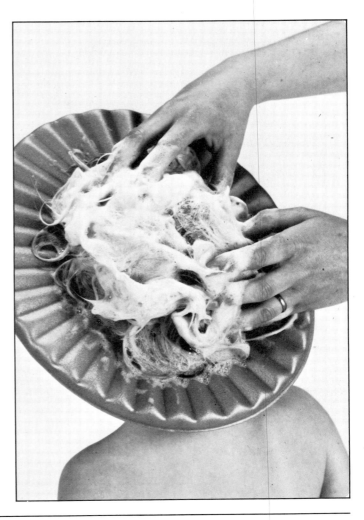

WASHING CHILDREN'S HAIR

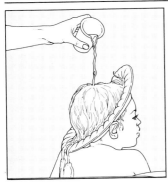

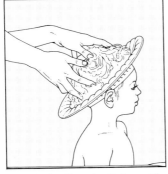

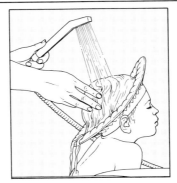

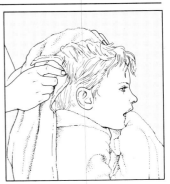

1. Carefully check temperature of water. Remember young skins are sensitive to heat and what feels only warm to an adult may be painfully hot to a child (85° to 90°F – 29° to 30°C – is about right).

2. Wet hair with water. Put a small quantity of shampoo into the palm of your hand and gently massage all over the scalp and hair.

3. You can use a shampoo shield to avoid irritating drips. Then, thoroughly rinse out all the soap making sure you rinse under shield.

4. Blot hair with a towel to remove surplus water. Make sure hair is quite dry.

Conditioning

Hair has to be in good condition to look good, so it is not surprising that manufacturers have found conditioners to be very good business. These days, many women rely on them heavily. Hair that is shoulder length or longer needs extra care to keep it in good condition. As well as having the ends trimmed regularly, conditioning will make it easier to comb through after shampooing. Short hair, too, often requires a great deal of conditioning.

Conditioners are just as important for men as they are for women and using them should not be thought of as something undesirable or unmanly — they should be applied as a matter of course after each shampooing.

Hair conditioners

While shampoos remove the oily film on the hair, conditioners help to counteract the effects of de-greasing. They will make the hair more manageable, elastic and glossy. There are thousands of different types on the market . . . and quite a few readily available in your own kitchen. The yolk of an egg, for example, has long been used as an after-shampoo pack to lend 'body' to the hair. So has beer, which can be poured over the hair undiluted and left, or rinsed off with warm water. Beer is known to be a good setting agent. A tablespoon of vinegar added to a pint of warm water will give the hair more elasticity and allow it to be combed more easily. The vinegar produces a slightly acid shield which is essential in well-conditioned hair. A rinse with a tablespoon of malt vinegar is particularly good for dry, brittle hair, as well as hair that has been bleached and tinted.

One advantage of using a conditioner is that it can make hair less fly-away. The conditioner coats the hair with a protective film that helps to reduce static electricity.

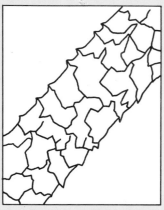

Before conditioning the outside of the hair shaft can look ragged, with the cuticles lifted. This makes it difficult to run a comb easily through the hair and leads to tangling.

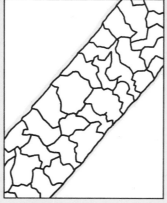

A conditioner will deposit a very fine wax-like film over each hair, helping to smooth down the cuticles. This invisible protective coating makes the hair more easy to handle.

As each hair is separated, there is less friction; the hair combs more easily and, as the coating smoothes the roughened hair shaft, it not only looks sleeker and shinier, but is less likely to tangle.

Usually, the application of conditioner is quick and easy: after shampooing and rinsing, a little conditioner is worked into the hair and combed through. It will be most effective if the hair has been blotted dry first. The conditioner is then left on the hair for a minute or so before it is rinsed off with plenty of warm water to get rid of any trace of surface stickiness. Many conditioners have been specially formulated for dry, normal or oily hair; for example, a conditioner that contains a coconut oil as one of its ingredients will probably be designed for dry and brittle hair, whereas lemon is identified with oily hair treatments because of its astringent properties.

A straightforward conditioner may help to keep hair that is basically healthy in good shape, especially if it is used after every shampoo. More drastic measures may be needed for problem hair. If hair has become damaged – through perming, tinting, straightening, or even through any number of natural causes, such as sun, wind or salt water – it may need a special conditioner that can partly penetrate the hair shaft. Such conditioners often contain protein in liquid form, and they are meant to penetrate the hair shaft to build up its natural protein structure. This type of conditioner also makes the hair anti-static and coats the cuticle so that it becomes smoother and looks shinier.

There are many organically based treatments available for damaged or dehydrated hair, using plant rather than animal protein to help strengthen and moisturize the hair. These products, known as 'restructurants', remain in the hair through a period of shampooing and usually need only be applied every few weeks. Often hairdressers will provide such treatments as part of their service.

It is important to remember that these treatments are meant for the hair, not for the scalp.

Scalp conditioners

Treatment for the scalp will involve the use of heat and massage, as well as oil. Various scalp conditioning treatments are carried out by trichologists and hairdressers and all are designed to cause the tiny blood capillaries in the upper layers of the skin of the scalp to dilate. Sometimes a vegetable oil, such as olive oil, is warmed to 55°C (131°F) and then brushed on to the scalp. Other treatments involve a hot towel being tightly wrapped around the head. Massage is also used to improve the circulation of the blood to the scalp which in turn makes the sebaceous glands more active and encourages hair growth.

Scalp treatments, although sometimes messy, can be done at home. Any vegetable oil can be used, although

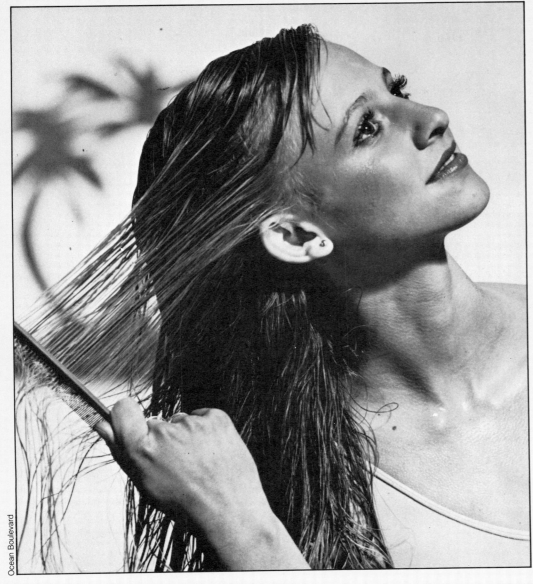

Ocean Boulevard

Most hair needs help to keep in good condition. Hair that is shoulder length or longer needs extra care to maintain it in top condition. As well as having the ends trimmed regularly, conditioning will make it easier to comb through after shampooing.

olive oil is highly recommended. After warming the oil in a pan, the hair should be parted and the oil applied to the entire length of the parting. Repeat this, making further partings along the entire head at 1-inch (2.5 centimetre) intervals, until the whole scalp is covered. After a massage with the tips of the fingers, lasting for at least five minutes for the best effect, wrap a hot towel around the head and leave it for half an hour or longer. To get a towel nice and hot, soak it in hot water and wring it out before winding it around the head. After the oil treatment, shampoo the hair and rinse it thoroughly.

Setting lotions, gels, mousses and foams are all designed to put the finishing touch to the hairstyle and often help it to stay in shape that little bit longer. Unfortunately, many setting lotions contain alcohol and plasticizers to 'fix' the hair and these can be harmful because of their drying effect.

Hairsprays also need to be carefully chosen. They should be lightweight and non-sticky in texture, with a fine even spray. The right spraying technique should be used: after shaking the can, it should be held some 8 to 10 inches (20 to 25 centimetres) away from the hair and, moving the can over the head from front to back, the hair should be sprayed lightly all over. If the can is held too close, the spray will build up in concentrated patches and make the hair feel heavy and coated.

Wet hair warning

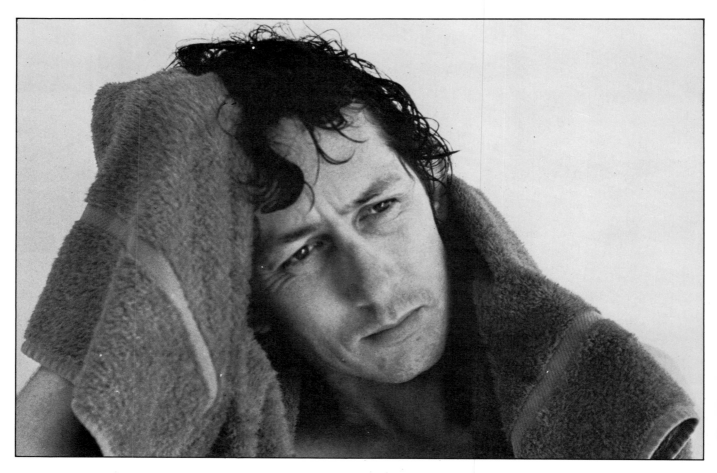

When hair is wet it is like elastic – easy to stretch. You can take a single healthy hair and, exerting a gradually increasing pull, stretch it to one-third longer than its natural length in the dry state. Healthy hair can withstand this treatment and then shrink back to its natural length without any harm being done.

Out-of-condition hair, however, cannot. It will break under undue tension. Even the best heads of hair are likely to have a percentage of hairs that are out of condition: the older growth almost ready to be shed, patches at the front or sides that have been more exposed to the elements and have 'weathered' or dried out, and even a few small tangles that will catch against a comb or brush. All of these weaknesses will be greatly increased when the hair is wet and in its most vulnerable state. So always take care when handling wet hair.

One thing you can do and that is: rinse your hair well with water containing a few drops of vinegar. This, in fact is exactly what our grandmothers used to do, and, even though your hair may be in excellent condition, if you live in a hard-water area it would be very wise to follow in their footsteps. Vinegar helps to give the hair a protective coating to form what is known as a 'liquid' shield that can remove the dulling film often left on the hair by hard water. Our ancestors probably knew as much as we do now about how to keep hair looking lovely and glossy.

As a preliminary to any drying process use a towel to blot dry, removing the excess moisture and leaving the hair in a damp rather than wet state. Then 'finger comb' — that is, simply run your fingers through your hair from scalp to ends to gently coax the hair into its natural fall and the lines in which it will be styled. This way you can ease out potential tangles before submitting the hair to a comb.

Do not use a brush on wet or damp hair. The action is too aggressive. Use a wide-toothed comb, starting the combing two or three inches (5 or 7.5 centimetres) from the tips of the hair and gradually working up towards the roots to ensure the hair lies smoothly. Now it can be left to dry naturally or with the aid of heat.

The most popular method of getting damp hair dry is by using a hair dryer and brush to blow dry the hair. As the brush is going to be used simply to hold the hair in place under the hot air stream and not to force the hair into line, it is quite safe to switch from comb to brush at this point.

Problem hair

Almost any type of hair can be improved with proper care. Different degrees of oily or dry hair will respond to specially formulated shampoos and conditioners. The label on the bottle will usually state whether the product is suitable for dry or oily hair.

Ingredients, such as particles of protein tiny enough to cling to the hair, can give dry or porous hair additional body. Liquid protein is also known to be an excellent reconditioner of damaged hair. When applied, it actually becomes part of the hair itself, strengthening the hair shaft and smoothing the cuticle of the hair.

Many hair problems stem from improper care of the scalp. For example, you may think that you have a dry scalp when you are actually suffering from a failure to wash the scalp often and thoroughly enough. When this happens, oil and dead skin are allowed to accumulate, forming a paste on the scalp that seals pores and oil glands. As a result, the hair appears to be dry, because the oil is prevented from flowing down the shafts. The solution is usually to shampoo the hair at least twice a week, brushing it daily with a soft brush so the oil is distributed along the entire length of the hair.

PROBLEMS	REMEDIES
Oily hair Your hair is oily if, three days after shampooing, you run your fingers over the scalp, press your fingertips firmly on a tissue and greasy fingerprints show up. If a set will not hold, hair is unmanageable or looks lank with strands clinging together, it is also very likely that the problem is oily hair. The same condition applies if the colour looks drab because dust is sticking to the hair.	You can wash excessively oily hair as often as necessary – daily, if you like. If the scalp is oily, apply a conditioner, but only to the hair itself. If you wash your hair very often, usually only one application of shampoo is needed each time. A mild shampoo is usually best, especially if you use it daily. Take care to rinse thoroughly. Wash your comb and brush in warm, soapy water at least once a week.
Dry hair Your hair is dry if, when you run fingertips along the length of your hair and gently rub ends between fingers and thumb, you hear a slight crackle and the hair feels rough. If the hair is fly-away and difficult to control, feels brittle or tends to tangle, a lack of natural oils is likely to be the problem.	Give your scalp a massage before you shampoo, using a deep penetrating conditioning treatment at least once a week if the hair is dry. You can use olive oil or other vegetable oils as a conditioning treatment, leaving it on overnight before shampooing the following morning. Commercial deep–conditioning treatments are usually applied after shampooing and should be left on for at least half an hour before rinsing.
Split ends You have split ends if the hair looks unruly, fuzzy at the tips, feels brittle and is difficult to set. Split ends occur mainly if the hair is dry and out of condition.	A good conditioning rinse will help prevent further damage. Split ends can cause the hair to tangle, but with the conditioner coating the hair shaft this problem is minimized. Rinse hair in cold water and avoid using hot rollers or hair dryers. Have the hair trimmed at the first opportunity.
Porous hair Your hair is porous if the hair feels spongy or greasy, especially at the tips. It is a condition caused by over-harsh or continuous bleaching or permanent waving.	Give porous hair a chance to recover by not having it permed or tinted for a while; cover the hair to shield it from extreme conditions and treat it as for split ends with a mild shampoo and regular conditioning.
Scurfy, dandruffy hair You have scurf (dandruff) if a fine sprinkling of whitish flakes show up when you brush or comb your hair. These are dry, powdery flakes of dead skin from the scalp. If larger oily, white flakes appear, it is a more advanced condition of dandruff which often goes with greasy hair.	Keep the scalp from getting too dry by frequent brushing, and massaging. Wash hair with an anti–dandruff shampoo, rinsing thoroughly to get rid of the flakes. Use a conditioner on hair and scalp to keep it moist. You usually need more conditioner in winter, when the skin tends to be drier. Avoid using hot hair dryers which can cause the scalp to dry out more; the more moist you can keep the scalp, the better.

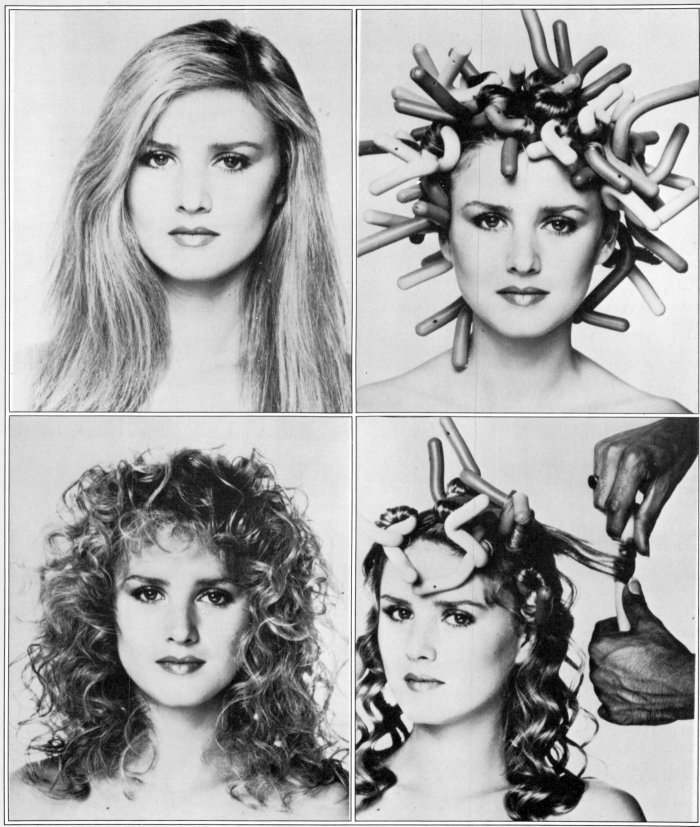

4
Drying and styling

Both drying and styling are very important for creating a good hair style. Care must be taken when handling the hair during these stages.

There are three different basic methods of drying and styling the hair after shampooing, each with its own variations. You can let your hair dry naturally; you can use a hair dryer, usually with a brush to style the hair; or you can use an electrical styling appliance. Your hairstyle will largely dictate what method you choose.

If your hair is very short, or you favour the wash-and-wear style that has been cut or permed to fall into a natural line, you can happily leave your hair to dry on its own accord after having combed it into place or pushed it into style with your fingers. Apart from being a time-saving and convenient way of drying your hair, it is also the kindest method of treating it – because any kind of heat applied to wet hair, no matter how carefully or how well-conditioned the hair, will be slightly drying to the hair's natural oils. However, with natural drying you are limited in the amount of styling effects you can realistically achieve. It is difficult to create any lift at the root or volume and movement in the style and you cannot get any movement unless it is already either naturally there or permed into the hair.

A way to produce the 'wild' look, with hair standing out from the head, is to plait (braid) your hair while it is damp in tiny strands all over the head. Leave to dry – overnight if necessary – and when the strands are unplaited (unbraided) you have a tiny zig-zag crimped effect. Go one step on and thread very fine ribbons through the plaits (braids) and you have a colourful dreadlock style to wear while you wait for your hair to dry.

One of the more unusual ways of setting the hair is, in fact, by using ribbons or fabric strips, similar to the old-fashioned rag-curlers method, and long bendy foam curlers which can be twisted into the hair to create waves and curls. Although not as easy to use as electrical styling gadgets, these curlers do have the benefit of being kind to the hair and are useful to use if your hair is not in the best condition and you want to give it a rest from heat setting.

RAG CURLING YOUR HAIR

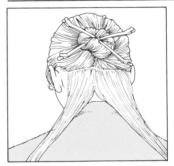

1. Start with the back sections, using clips to keep the hair you are not working on out of the way.

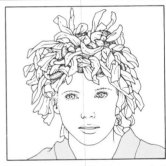

2. Start from the tip of the strand of hair and roll up to roots, then bend both ends of curler towards the centre of wound hair.

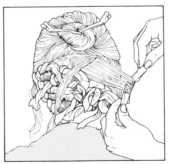

3. When you have put all your hair in curlers neatly and securely you can speed up drying process with hand-held dryer.

4. To check, undo one of the longest curlers to see if the hair is dry and curly enough.

Facing page: Bendy foam curlers can transform straight hair into curls. The technique is simple and effective because the curlers are smooth and kind to the hair.

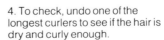

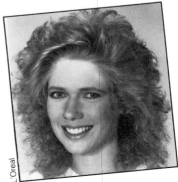

L'Oreal

Hair dryers

DRYING LONG HAIR

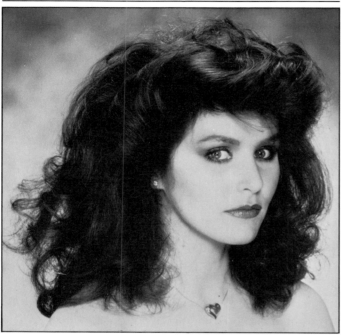

Henara Henna

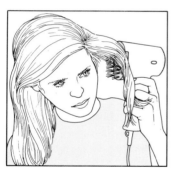

1. For drying and styling long, thick hair, choose a hand-held dryer that offers a high temperature and maximum air flow for efficient drying, and a choice of styling attachments to give movement and curl.

2. Use the dryer at maximum power to semi-dry hair. Then switch to low power and attach a vent brush with wide-spaced bristles to brush through the under layers of hair and create fullness.

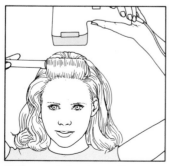

3. Change to the dryer with a nozzle attachment for a concentrated hot-air stream for setting the top meshes of hair around the crown into curl and wave movement.

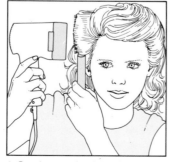

4. Continue around the sides of the head and, as the hair dries, switch to the low temperature setting to finish the curling process and give a longer-lasting set.

If you use a hair dryer you have the choice of a hand-held or a hood dryer. You will use the hand-held dryer if you are going to blow dry your hair – that is, use a brush to move individual sections of hair into the direction you want them to dry, put curve and movement into the ends and lift at the crown, while directing a stream of hot air to follow the brush movements as you dry the hair section by section. You can use a hood dryer if you set your hair in rollers or pin-curls. This is a head-enveloping dome with transparent plastic sides and front visor, which blasts out hot air all round the head.

With both methods you have to be careful not to expose the hair to too much direct heat which, if excessive, could be harmful.

Using a hand-held dryer requires a certain skill and patience, as it takes quite a time to ensure that the under layers of hair are thoroughly dry before starting on the top layers. But once you have mastered the art of blow drying, it is a technique that is just right for youthful, fashionable styles, encouraging the hair to fall into its own natural line for a good-looking set.

Most people own a hand-held dryer, which is the most popular of all electrical hair care appliances. Originally it was simply used for drying the hair after it had been set in rollers or pin-curls. Then in the early 1970s the fashion for simple cut-and-blow-dry styling hit the hairdressing world and do-it-yourself hairstyling took off in a big way. The hand-held dryer became more than just a method of drying your hair; it became a styling system that allowed you to build body, direction and movement into the hair at the same time as you were drying it.

The basic pistol-grip style of hand-held dryer evolved into sleeker, smarter lines; dual-power and multiple-heat models, travel styles and semi-professional implements were developed into sophisticated and economically priced hair care aids for the home market.

The type of hand-held dryer you use should depend on both your hair and the type of style you want to achieve. But a basic rule is to choose a dryer that feels well balanced, comfortable to hold and light enough in weight to avoid making the arm ache. Variable heat settings that range from a cool 500 watts to a high-powered 1500 watts and different strengths of airflow will cope with a range of hairstyles.

Most dryers have a detachable nozzle that provides the choice of a wide spread of hot air for general drying and for coping with wide meshes of hair or for concentrating the air flow into a controlled stream for smooth and sleek contoured curves and curls.

Generally speaking, if you have long, thick hair that you wear straight, a high temperature, maximum airflow dryer will be the most efficient. Start by drying your hair with your head down, so the hair falls away from the scalp. This makes sure the under layers are completely dry and helps to provide lift at the roots to give the appearance of more body and fullness in the finished style.

If your hair is long, fine and fly-away, a dryer with a less forceful airflow is best because the hair will be less inclined to blow about and tangle as you dry it. For medium to short hair that is well cut and falls into place easily, a dryer with a wide, flat nozzle to dry large sections of hair quickly will be most suitable. If you want to mould the fringe (bangs) or sides to flick backwards or curve away from the main line of the hair, use the nozzle attachment to control the airflow and confine its spread to the area you are working on.

Start blow drying on the under section of your hair first, having pinned the upper layers out of the way on top of the crown. Working from the nape of the neck, lift a section of hair with the brush close to the scalp, gently easing it away from the head. Direct the flow of air from the dryer on the top half of the brush. This way it deflects the stream of hot air and discourages a direct jet of heat on the hair. Never let the dryer come closer than 6 inches (15 centimetres) to your hair and keep it moving so that direct heat never plays on one section of hair for more than a few seconds at a time.

Direct the air flow from the roots towards the tips, to smooth down the cuticles and encourage the hair to fall in its natural line. Keep twisting the brush to create curve at the ends and fullness at the roots. Work round the side sections in the same way, then unpin the upper layers and dry them. Finish by incorporating the under and upper layers into one and, section by section, smoothing the hair into the desired line.

Variations on this basic drying technique will create differences in style. A large brush produces volume and curve and a slimmer brush produces movement and curl. Flick-up (flipped-up) curls, feathered-back fringes (bangs) and sleekly styled bobs can all be easily achieved with patience and skill that comes from practising different blow drying techniques.

Work methodically over the head section by section. If any part of the hair dries before you have got the volume or movement you want, dampen it down with a light spraying of water. Also, it is beneficial to begin the drying process by applying a lotion, made especially for use in blow drying. It will help protect the condition of your hair as well as give a better finish and longer-lasting setting effect.

A hood dryer is the ideal method if you like the traditional and longer-lasting hairset. It takes a lot longer for the hair to dry, because the heat has to penetrate through the thick, damp meshes of hair wrapped round rollers or formed into tight pin-curls (added to the time it takes to set the hair in rollers and curls). But the hair can be moulded into flattering shapes that do stay in place until the next shampoo.

DRYING SHORT HAIR

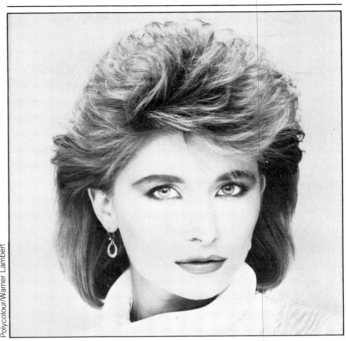

Polycolour/Warner Lambert

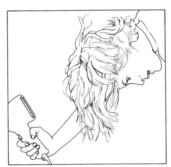

1. A blow dryer and brush attachment will quickly give bounce and crown height to short hair. Work quickly, keeping the dryer and brush moving all the time to avoid risk of heat damage.

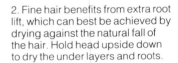

2. Fine hair benefits from extra root lift, which can best be achieved by drying against the natural fall of the hair. Hold head upside down to dry the under layers and roots.

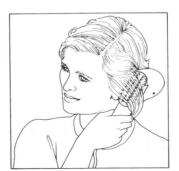

3. Switch dryer to a low setting and add the radial (round) brush attachment to put volume and curve into the sides of the hair.

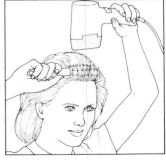

4. A brush and dryer, on a low temperature setting and with the concentrating nozzle attached, is used to give lift at the crown and on the front section.

45

*Rollers and pin-curls*_____

Roller setting is the oldest method of hair styling. It goes back to ancient Egyptian times when canes were used, through to its heyday in the 1960s when tin cans were called into service to produce the large diameter curve required to produce the volume needed for beehive and bouffant hair styles, and on to today when rollers tend more often than not to be heated, for speed and convenience.

But whatever their size, the principle of roller setting is the same. Wet hair is wound round the roller, left to dry naturally or with the help of heat, so it is set into a curve and then gently unwound from the roller. The smaller the diameter of the roller, the smaller the curl. The larger the diameter of the roller, the larger the curl. If using heat to dry the hair, once the hair is dry, allow the rollers to cool before removing gently and finger wind the curls back into place to ensure the hair is completely cool before starting to comb out. This will give a firmer set.

There are many different types of curler, one of the most popular being a wire spiral covered with nylon mesh and, in some cases, featuring a radial (round) brush-like insert with bristles that protrude through the mesh to grip the hair. Another popular type is the smooth cylinder of plastic which has an almost magnetic attraction to wet hair. Holes in the roller enable it to be pierced with hairpins and held safely in place. Foam type rollers also provide good gripping properties and are gentle on the hair – very important if your hair is not in tip-top condition.

Rollers can be used on wet or dry hair, but in the latter case you will probably need to use a little hair spray or setting lotion to reinforce the curl. Be careful in your choice of pins to anchor the roller in place. They need to be sharp enough to penetrate the roller, but should not be so spiky that they run the risk of tearing at or damaging fragile hair. Be careful how you use them, too. Ease them through the hair and roller rather than stabbing them in roughly.

Whatever type of roller is used, the setting method remains constant. The hair must be wound smoothly and at a firm, even tension, without stretching or placing any strain on the hair. If the wet hair is wound too tightly, it is in a stretched state and, as the hair dries, it shrinks back to its normal length, causing pull at the hair roots and the risk of breakage or damage.

The strand of hair that is wound round the roller should be lifted from the rest of the hair and held at right angles to the scalp. It is combed smooth and then wound on the roller until the roller reaches the scalp immediately over the hair roots to produce lift and bounce. If the hair is wound at anything less than a right angle, a flattening result will occur at the roots and the style will lack volume and movement.

Set the crown section of the hair first and then the back, sides and front. Do not take up too much hair on to each

ROLLER SETTING YOUR HAIR

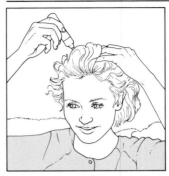

1. Towel dry hair well and apply the setting agent. There is an increasing variety of agents to choose from, for example some have added colour.

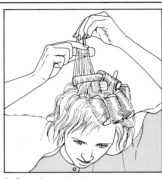

2. Start from the front and work backwards. Wind ends of hair round the curler first – keep the ends smooth.

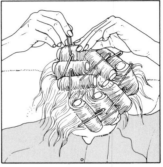

3. Secure the roller firmly with a pin. The tighter the roller the better the set. Do remember, however, that too much pull on the hair can damage it.

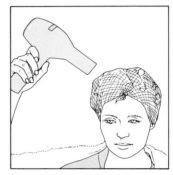

4. When all the rollers are in put on a net and dry with a hand-held dryer or hood-dryer.

roller and, if you want to reinforce the style with setting lotion, apply just a little to each section of hair as you wind the hair round.

With roller setting it is easy to vary your hair style according to the number of rollers used and the size of rollers chosen. You can combine curls and waves, create soft curves or lots of movement as you wish, to suit your length and texture of hair.

Pin-curls

Hand-in-hand with roller setting goes that other long-established technique – pin-curls. This is the best method for very short hair, especially the side and back sections that might not be long enough to wind easily on rollers. It also works well for styles that call for close-to-the-head waves.

There are two basic ways of winding pin-curls – either

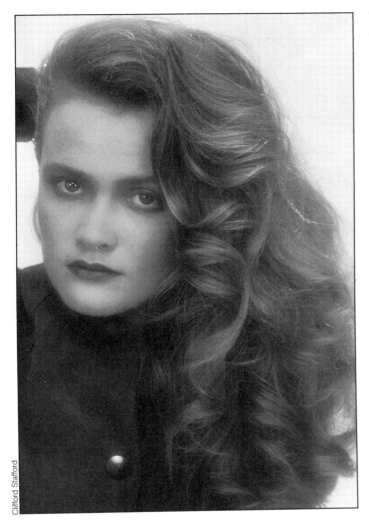

Clifford Stafford

TWO STYLES USING ROLLERS

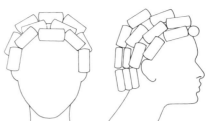

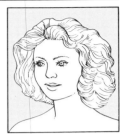

If your layered shoulder-length hair is fine, set it on medium to small rollers to achieve this soft wavey hairstyle. However, if you have a head of coarse curly hair, set it in large rollers, in order to create the same effect. The rollers have been wound 'brick' fashion, away from the hairline up to the crown, and then vertically towards the middle, from the crown to the nape of the neck.

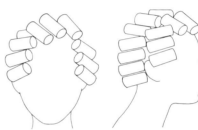

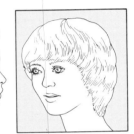

To achieve this wavey style on slightly shorter hair, put the rollers in at an angle to the hairline and forward on to the face. The back rollers are set horizontally and down, towards the nape. So that the fringe does not have a sectioned look use one large roller to set it. When the rollers are dry remove them and gently brush the hair forward, onto the face.

flat against the head or as an open curl that is rolled into a loop shape and gives a similar effect to using a roller. Either way, only small strands of hair can be wound at a time and the method is only successful with short hair. It is not effective with frizzy hair.

Flat pin-curls are used to create waves and movement close to the head. The diameter of the curl determines the size of the wave, so the smaller the curl, the tighter the wave, and the larger the diameter, the softer the wave or the looser the curl. Tramline (slip) waving effect can be achieved by combining ordinary pin-curling with reverse pin-curling. That is when one row of curls is wound in one direction and the row below is wound to follow the opposite direction and so on, alternating row by row down the sides and back of the hair.

The open or stand-up pin-curl gives more volume to a style. The section of hair is combed out at right angles to the scalp and winding begins at the end, turning the curl under and anchoring it firmly at the scalp with a grip (bobby pin) or clip.

Pin-curl setting is a traditional method of styling, as is finger waving – which simply means pushing the damp hair into a wave shape and fixing with a clip until the hair dries. These methods have been used in one form or another for centuries. They have been largely superseded by electrical hair setting and styling appliances, such as heated rollers, curling tongs, crimping irons and hot brushes. Where hair is fragile or in poor condition these former methods provide a gentler and safer method of setting than the latter. However, the modern appliances may prove to be more effective setting and styling methods. This is provided that the pins used to secure the rollers have blunt, ball-point ends rather than sharp spikes than can tear delicate hair; provided that the rollers are not wound too tightly, putting unnecessary tension on the hair; and provided the set is not 'baked' into place.

Electrical styling appliances

Electrical styling appliances comprise the heated rollers, hot brushes, tongs, wand stylers and crimping irons. They are useful for creating special styling effects – curls, waves, crinkles, movement or a smooth, sleek line. Make sure that there is no risk of the hair overheating through too-long exposure to tongs and irons. It is not advisable to use these types of appliance too frequently on hair that is in poor or brittle condition.

Hot brushes, electric curling tongs, styling wands and crimping irons should be used on freshly dried hair to avoid the risk of damage from the pulling action on wet hair that is necessary with these methods of styling. However, if you take into account the protective measures previously described, you can style confidently and successfully.

Take the utmost care with whatever method of heat drying you use. Do not subject the hair to it too frequently, because it can have a bad effect on its condition, drying out the natural moisture and reducing the hair's elasticity, eventually weakening it. When you have time and the and the opportunity, let your hair dry naturally and use your electrically heated styling aids on hair that is dry rather than wet and fragile.

Heated rollers

Maintaining a well-kept hairstyle has never been easier, thanks to all the styling aids around today. Most noticeable must be the heated roller that revolutionized the hair care appliance market in the mid-1960s, allowing a quicker setting and drying method and an easy way to boost a failing hairset.

The principle of the electrically heated roller is simplicity itself. The acrylic casing contains a special heat-retaining liquid and when the roller is set on an electrically heated metal rod the wax also heats up and stays hot for 10 to 15 minutes, which is long enough to set hair wound round the roller into curl.

These rollers come in sets with different sizes for use on short and long sections of hair. A large set will have two dozen rollers in three sizes, an average set will have between 16 and 20 rollers in two sizes and you can even get small travel sets holding six or so rollers.

From the early days there have been several modifications in design: they have been improved with smoother teeth to grip the hair without risk of tearing or damaging it and some incorporate conditioning lotion to help prevent heat damage and protect the hair. They are popular because they can give a swift, effortless change of style and a variety of looks. You can achieve a curly, wavy or bouncy style depending on the size of rollers used. Timing also helps to create styling changes and how long you leave the rollers in the hair determines how tight or loose the curl will be. Remove them after three minutes or so when they are still warm and you get less curl, more of a curved shape. Leave them in until cold for 15 minutes or longer and the hair is set into firm curl.

If you choose to dry your hair with heated rollers, remove as much moisture as possible by blot drying with a towel. On hair that is very fine, has been bleached, or is in any way fragile, it is worth either wrapping a tissue around each roller or using a perming end-paper on the tips of each section of hair. This gives a little protection and avoids direct heat being applied to the hair. When the rollers have cooled, remove them gently and finger wind the curls back into place to ensure the hair is completely cool before you start combing out.

Electric stylers

The most versatile of these styling appliances is the electric styler, which is a combination of hand-held dryer and – through a series of styling attachments – a hot brush, hot comb and wand. The attachments are designed to fit on to the nozzle of the dryer, so the hot air

A heated curling brush can change straight shoulder-length hair to a style which curls under at the ends to frame the face in soft feminine curls. It is a styling technique that is easy to master and can instantly transform an everyday style into a pretty party look.

48

streams through between the bristles of the brush or the teeth of the comb, or along vents in the wand.

By varying the temperature setting on the dryer and spreading or concentrating the air flow and controlling its power, you can create the most beneficial drying and styling techniques for your individual requirements. Different hair lengths, textures and styles will call for different treatments, and the latest types of electric stylers should provide the hair drying technique that will suit you best.

The hot brush works a bit like the heated roller and can be used for long or short hair for quick and easy styling, whether to add waves, curls or curves – or even to straighten out over-curly hair. The metal barrel of the brush transmits heat through the bristles to help coax the hair into curl. Some brushes come with interchangeable bristles to provide short bristles for styling short hair and setting tighter curls and longer bristles to give better control of long hair, providing more movement and volume where needed.

Use the brush to give volume and bounce, especially to root section, to put wave movement into long hair, and to provide lift at the crown on short hair. The larger the radius of the brush, the looser the curls and the larger the wave movements will be.

Tongs and wands (curling irons)

Similar devices are hot tongs and electric styling wands (curling irons), both modern-day versions of the old metal curling tongs that used to be heated up on the stove. The smooth, heated barrel makes them less inclined to cause tangles and so on long hair they are often better than the hot brush. They can provide tighter, ringlet-style curls, make waves or be used literally to iron out frizz to give better controlled curls. They come in a choice of barrel sizes to give tight or loose curls and some have holes in the barrel and a water reservoir in the handle to produce steam to fix the curl more effectively.

When winding hair round styling tongs, start from the tips and wind towards the roots, stopping just short of the scalp to avoid any chance of burning your head with the hot iron.

Another version of heated tongs is the crimping iron, which consists of two flat surfaces with V-shaped indentations. Place a section of hair between the two surfaces, clamp the iron shut for a few seconds, and a series of V-shaped waves are crimped into the hair. Treat the meshes like this from root area to tips and you get a wild-looking mane of hair standing out from the head.

Alternatively, you can use the wand for small curls and more controlled waving techniques. It is also useful for creating smooth lines and combatting frizzy hair problems, and for putting a soft curve into the tips of the hair.

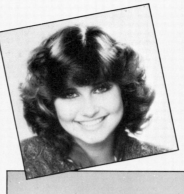

Top: *Styling tongs (curling irons) can be used to create a variety of effects, for example, face-framing waves.*

Below: *A tumbling mass of ringlet curls. There are different sizes of tongs (irons) to give tight curls or loose waves and they are used to best effect on hair that has been towel-dried and is barely damp. You then avoid 'boiling' the hair, so damage is less likely.*

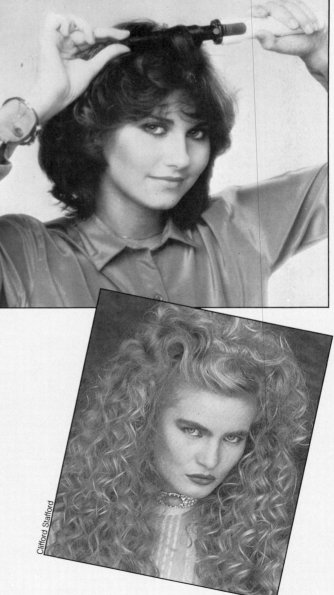

Clifford Stafford

49

Holding your hair in place

All these methods of setting can be used with setting lotion to reinforce the strength and staying-power of the style. Apply after shampooing to towel-dried hair as each strand is curled or rollered – but make sure the hair is thoroughly dry before unwinding.

There are many different types of setting lotion, some of which are expensive. To save money, use some left-over beer as a setting lotion. It will not only prove very effective; it is also very good for the hair.

Another way to preserve your set is with hairspray, especially if the weather is windy or a little damp. This is applied after the hair has been styled by spraying from a distance of 12 inches (30 centimetres) in a fine, even mist all over the head. Do not use too much – and brush it out at bedtime to avoid a build-up that can leave the hair looking dull. Hairsprays come in aerosol can form, which gives a fine, evenly dispersed spray, or in a pump-activated bottle or can, which does not give quite such a fine spray but which is considered better for the environment because it does not pose a threat to the earth's ozone layer.

Mousses and gels

Many hairstyles seem to defy the law of gravity and, if this is the case, a styling mousse can be invaluable. The mousse can be applied to wet or dry hair and, once combed through, will allow the hair to be slicked or scrunched into shape. It can also be used in between shampoos to help moisturize and condition the hair when it has become a bit lifeless. After applying on dry hair, simply blow dry it back in shape until the next shampoo.

Styling gels are also useful in helping to make the hair more manageable. Some are formulated with conditioning ingredients, adding fullness and body without making the hair stiff and sticky. Combed through damp hair and simply allowed to dry, the gel will help create a wet look. It can also be finger styled to give the hair more volume.

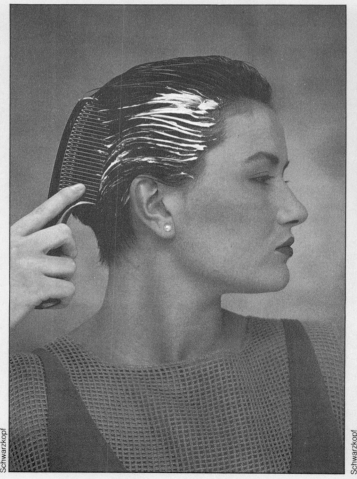
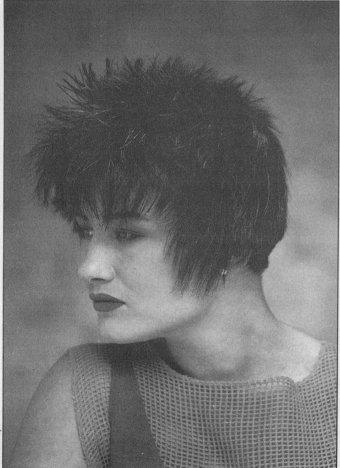

Above: *Mousses and gels are the ideal setting aid for tousled, spiky styles.*

50

Rescuing tired hair

With all the modern aids that are available for home hair care, shampooing, setting and styling are usually quickly and easily done with the minimum of fuss, but nonetheless these processes still take time to carry out. Often there simply is not the time, because of a sudden date or unexpected appointment. Or maybe you were caught in a shower and your hairstyle is a mess.

Then it is a case of taking emergency measures to salvage a ruined hairdo or to pep up a drooping set.

Probably the best known 'rescue operation' is the dry shampoo as a quick way to counteract oily hair. Dry shampoo is a powder – usually finely ground orris root or talc – that is sprinkled through the hair, worked gently in with fingertips – especially around the root area which will be the greasiest part – and then left for five minutes.

During this time the powder will absorb some of the excess grease and, as you brush out the powder, so you take some of the grease with it. You have to brush very thoroughly to remove the powder, but even then it is not really possible to remove every trace and you usually end up with a dull and filmy deposit on the hair. For this reason, dry shampooing is a method best suited to blond and light brown shades of hair rather than dark brown and brunette colouring, where the white film will show up more clearly.

However, for blonds in an emergency it can be a useful technique . . . and if you have no dry shampoo to hand, turn to the kitchen cupboard and use cornflour (corn starch) which is a close substitute.

For brunettes having to cope with the sudden situation of greasy hair, a better method is to try and tackle the root of the problem – literally – and clean up the scalp with a little eau de cologne or witch hazel. Make partings in the hair and gently dab along their length with a cotton wool pad soaked in the cologne or mildly astringent witch hazel to remove some of the grease.

Another method that can help remove grease is to cover a hairbrush with an absorbent cloth, such as cheesecloth, butter muslin or a soft cotton, or push strips of the fabric between the rows of bristles and brush gently to get rid of surface dust and remove some of the grease which will be absorbed into the cloth.

Tired and limp hair

You can boost a tired hairset with a revitalizing roller routine. Just comb and part your hair as for normal setting and dampen each piece of hair very lightly with quick-drying setting lotion or hairspray before winding it on to the roller. Leave until quite dry – usually between five to 10 minutes depending on the length of your hair – then brush out and style as usual.

Alternatively, you can give a quick set to a style by using a gel. If your hair is fairly short it is quite effective to

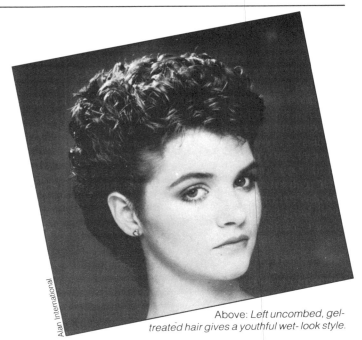

Above: *Left uncombed, gel-treated hair gives a youthful wet-look style.*

apply the gel, comb through into the line of style you want and leave. This gives the hair a wet look which is usually preferable to having a limp-looking tired hairstyle. Another rescue operation for lank locks, if your hair is medium to long, is to comb the hair back off the sides of the face and catch it back with grips (bobby pins) or tie it into a ponytail so you do not have the rat's tail effect of hair hanging loose around your face.

Quick colour

If the colour of your hair is a problem and you have not had time to get your roots retouched and there is noticeable growth, you can try some camouflage work with fantasy colour. If you wear a hairstyle with a parting, choose a gold or silver spray-on or paint-on temporary colourant and concentrate on putting little flecks of colour along the parting and the occasional streak through the hair to help it blend in. If you wear a hairstyle without a parting, it is easier to disguise the roots with some judicious back-combing to make the hair stand away from the head so the root section is less noticeable.

Naturally white hair or a bleached ash-blond colour can often suffer from unattractive yellowing, especially at the front where smoke from a cigarette can cause nicotine staining. If you have not got the time to rectify the problem with an ash rinse, you can try a quick disguise with spray-on colouring. Again use gold or silver, whichever is closest to the colour of your hair, and cover up the offending patch. If that does not work too well, go for a dramatic effect and spray a bold streak of contrasting colour through your hair to detract from the patchiness and to draw attention to yourself!

51

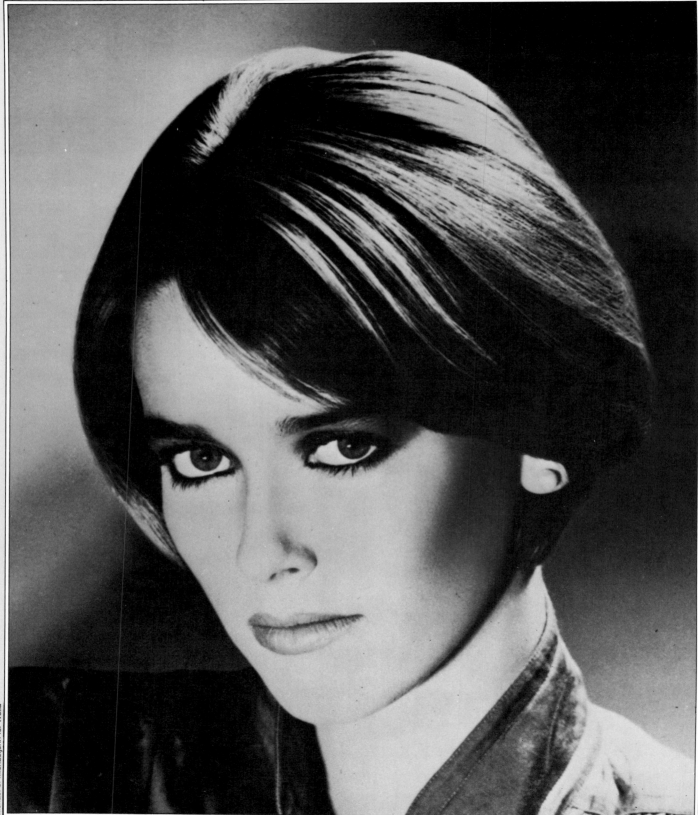

5

Cuts and cutting

It takes years to train a stylist to become technically proficient at cutting hair. A great many never really make it – and often it is not only because the technique is lacking. Cutting hair the way that suits a client requires a stylist to be an artist who must be perfectly in tune with the fashion requirements of the day. He or she must also have a 'feel' and understanding of the client's life style, as well as the technical ability to work within the limitations imposed by the quality of the hair itself. It is not surprising that hair cutting has become a speciality in its own right rather than being seen as a preliminary to further hair treatments, such as perming or colouring.

Thirty years ago the hairdressing industry was very different to what it is today. Those were the days of the hairdresser whose creations were often so elaborate that no woman would dare to imagine she could accomplish anything like it herself at home. It proved to be a bad policy for the craft as many young women were staying away. They knew it wouldn't be a question of a simple cut, but that their hair would have to be 'dressed'. Usually, this meant having to wait for a week before the next appointment until the hair could be washed and dressed again.

The young and trendy would run a mile rather than subject themselves to a pair of scissors, so wild and long-flowing hair became the order of the day in the 1960s. It was the age of Brigitte Bardot and the Rolling Stones; an age that would no longer tolerate the constraints of an out-of-date hairdressing industry.

'It's the cut that counts', said Vidal Sassoon more than 20 years ago, and acting on those few words, he went on to revolutionize the hairdressing business worldwide. Now it is accepted that a hairdresser's priority is to get the cut as near perfect as possible, even before other treatments such as perms or highlights are considered.

Sassoon also preached that there can be no hard and fast rules about cutting hair. Each client sets the stylist a different set of problems. Whether the hair is thick or thin, coarse or fine, curly or straight – a haircut can only be judged a success after it has performed well in the rigours of a particular environment. Secretaries, ballet dancers, housewives and models will all have very different ideas as to what constitutes a good haircut. Sitting behind a desk, the secretary may well be able to keep long, flowing hair unruffled, whereas the young mother with kids in tow who constantly rushes in and out of the house will only be happy with an easy-care, no-fuss bob. Medium to long hair may be ideal for the model in giving scope to change the style instantly, but it can be a positive nuisance to the nurse who must keep hair out of the way.

Age, height and figure

Age, height and type of figure will play a major part in deciding your hair cut. If you have always fancied a hairstyle like one of those film idols from the past, think twice! It is wrong to think of your hair in isolation. It is no use attempting a Marilyn Monroe style unless you too have the voluptuous lips, soft baby-like cheeks and sensuous hooded eyes. You will need to have the classic fine features to attempt the type of looks made fashionable by Grace Kelly in the fifties . . . even if your hair is already shoulder-length and you don't have a fringe (bangs). And, if your hair is dark, thick and curly like Elizabeth Taylor's, you will still need to have the flawless complexion and glowing eyes to achieve a similarly dramatic effect to the one she creates.

Proportion is everything in beauty and your hairstyle is no exception. If you are tall and slim, for example, a short haircut that lies close to the head will only serve to accentuate your height, making your head look tiny and out of proportion with the rest of the body. A fuller, longer style will create a more balanced effect and give a softer impression. A chopped-off, square-looking style is the wrong choice when you are tall with a full figure. This type of hairstyle only serves to deflect attention away from the head to the body – the last thing you may wish if your shape is less than perfect. Instead, a soft, full hairstyle that shows up your best facial features will be a good choice. A full hairstyle may 'dwarf' someone who is tiny, giving an unflattering top-heavy look. For a tiny body, a neat and tiny haircut is usually most flattering.

Face shape

A hairdresser must work on the head rather like a sculptor: the finished hairstyle should look good from every angle. This means that, as well as having to consider the type of hair and way it grows, the stylist will carefully analyse the shape of your face and neck. Styling effects can be used to enhance the most attractive features and to help camouflage any facial flaws.

Just because a style is fashionable is never a good enough reason to choose it, because hair cannot be regarded in isolation. A long neck is elegant, but sometimes it can be too long for your height. If this is the case, avoid short styles or hair piled on the crown. On the other hand, hair taken to the top of the head and pulled off the face will make a short neck look thinner. An excessively rounded forehead may be flattered with a helmet-cut fringe (bowl-cut bangs) that smoothly covers the eyebrows. A hairstyle that hugs the face, with soft waves especially at the chin line and without a fringe (bangs), will draw attention away from a receding chin line, whereas fringes (bangs) are effective in distracting attention from a heavy chin.

In fact a fringe is probably the most effective part of a hairstyle in helping to emphasize an attractively shaped face or disguising a less than perfect one. There are so many ways a fringe can be worn. It can be a half fringe, brushed slantwise across the forehead, a full heavy fringe to totally cover the forehead and draw attention to the eyes, or a wispy, sparse fringe that can soften a severe hairstyle. It can completely alter a hairstyle or create a new look, but it does need careful alteration. Because a fringe is such a prominent part of a hairstyle, it is immediately noticeable if it has been badly cut and is usually the first part of the hair to look out of shape and in need of cutting. Also, on hair that tends towards greasiness a fringe can often look limp and unattractive, so it needs to be well cared for to look its most effective.

As a rough guide, facial shapes usually fall in one of five categories: oval, oblong, round, square, triangular or heart-shaped.

Oval shape

The oval-shaped face is considered to be near perfect, simply because its width and length ratio are thought to be ideal. If you are lucky enough to have an oval face, the hairdresser will probably select a style designed to flatter this ideal contour. Any hair length is suitable, although very short or chin-length can look most attractive. Having an oval-shaped face does not, of course, guarantee that your features will be flawless to match. Even so, the stylist can use plenty of tricks of the trade to disguise imperfections. For example, a full hairstyle will help balance a large full mouth and a loose, wavy style will soften sharp features. If the nose is prominent, the stylist

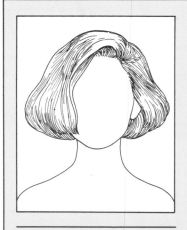

OVAL

If you are constantly coverting other people's hairstyles, but can never pluck up enough courage to try them out yourself, cut out your face shape from an old passport photograph. When you have decided which shape you face is, place it over the appropriate blanked out faces shown here. There are four categories of face shape provided - oval, oblong round and square.

Not every face is flawless: even an oval face, which is generally considered to be the perfect shape, may contain some flaws. Almost any hair style will suit an oval face which has balanced features, but remember that your choice of hairstyle is governed by your hair-type, so you should consider your hairline and the length and texture of your hair before you decide on a particular hair cut. The picture above left shows a light, graduated bob which is full at the sides and therefore shows off the perfect oval shape of the model's face.

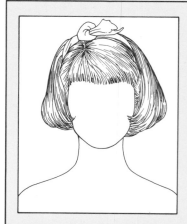

OBLONG

These are various techniques that can be used to substantially reduce the length of a long face. One such method is to have a full fringe (bangs), which appears to 'cut the face in half', giving the illusion of a shorter and broader shape. Hair should ideally be kept at jaw length, and preferably off the face with plenty of volume at ear level. If the hair is long and straight it will automatically emphasize the length of your face. If you are determined to have long hair, it is flattering to have a curl or gentle wave put in it. An asymmetrical hairstyle, easily achieved by a side-parting and a wave in the hair, gives an unbalanced look and therefore takes away from the length of the face and is recommended. The picture on the left shows a jaw length bob with a fringe. The bob is very full at ear level, which gives breadth to a long face. When the hair is lank or limp, before washing, draw hair off the face with clips to add width.

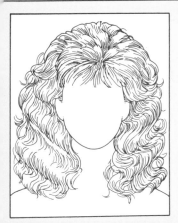

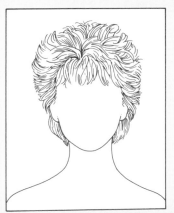

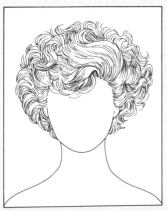

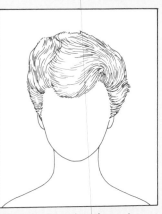

If you have curly hair, whether naturally curly or whether permed and waved, if you have short layers of hair on the top of your head and long layers at the back and sides, set 1 inch (2.5 centimetres) sections of your hair in heated rollers to achieve a mass of pretty curls. Use setting mousse or lotion when you are setting your hair so that, when dry, it keeps its shape, body and style.

A short casual hairstyle can be scrunch dryed, or blow dryed, to create this rough tousled look. Mousse or setting gel should be applied either before or after drying to achieve the soft effect on the fringe (bangs), as shown here. In order to lighten the total look from the front, it may need to be pointed or thinned.

This style is short at the back, but the layers at the top of the head have been kept long. The curl may be natural or can be achieved by permanent waving, heated rollers, curling brush or tongs (curling irons). Backcombing the layers may also successfully achieve the same effect. The hair shown here is fine.

The style shown here is most suitable for course hair. It is a neat, conventional style that has been swept across the head, and gives emphasis to the oval shaped face.

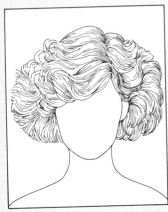

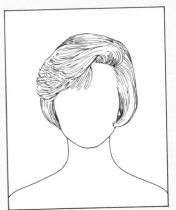

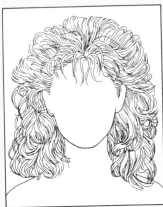

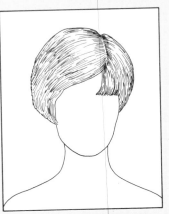

A long face needs to be framed by a full hairstyle. Here, the waved fringe (bangs), cut so that it sweeps over one side of the face, creates a shorter space between the eyes and lips. Also, allowing the ears to show gives an illusion of width to the face.

Another bob, this time with a long fringe (bangs), to give width to the eyebrows, and a graduated bottom line to leave weight at the ears and make the hair curve in from ears to chin level. This style is suitable for any texture of hair, and can be blow dryed or combed and left to dry naturally.

Occasionally, with good use of colour, curls, accessories and make-up, an off-the-face layered hairstyle - with width behind the ears, to frame the face - can look stunning, even on a long face if the face is 'shortened' by teasing long tendrils down over the forehead. With curly hair this style can be achieved by scrunch drying. For straight hair heated rollers are necessary.

This short asymmetrical style shows a mass of hair over the crown and forehead, framing the top half of the face, thus 'cutting the face in half'. This styling technique is complemented by the hair having been cut with a flat top so as not to elongate the face from the cheekbones downwards. The cut exhibits diagonal lines which further lessen the length of the face.

will avoid a centre parting which will seem to connect with the line of the nose and draw attention to it.

Oblong shape

An oblong face is longer than it is wide, with the cheeks, jaw and forehead more or less equal in width. To shorten the length, the hair can be cut to fall over the forehead or it can be used to build width around the side of the head. A soft style will break what could be a severe line and usually a loose, natural hair design, accented by natural waves or curl brushed on to the face rather than away from it, is most flattering.

Round shape

A round face is two-thirds as wide as it is long, with the cheeks the widest part of the face. The jawline and forehead taper gently. This can give a girlish look even to mature women. A style that is asymmetrical, for example, one that features a definite side parting or sweeps across one side of the forehead, will minimize the roundness. Framing the face and building up hair at the top of the head will create a more angular look and highlight the cheekbones. A round face should never have a full fringe (bangs), as this will emphasize the roundness of the lower face.

Square shape

A square face also has a width two-thirds or more of the length, but the forehead, jaw and cheeks are almost equally wide. A good haircut should soften the lines by giving the illusion of less width and more height. A full hairstyle at the cheek bones and temples, falling in soft lines from a side parting, will make the face appear rounder. Fringes (bangs) covering corners of the forehead will soften the abrupt angle of the hairline.

Triangular or heart-shape

A triangular face shape has wide cheek bones and a large forehead. Often the chin is pointed. This is also known as a heart-shaped face and the most flattering hairstyle will usually avoid width at the sides but not at the back of the neck. A medium-length bob with a full fringe (bangs) can help soften the contours and give a good balance to the face. Another variation is the 'inverted triangle', or pear-shaped, face. This needs a style that is widest at the temples and sufficiently built up off the forehead to compensate for a prominent jaw. The hair should be short or swept back off the face below the ears and long styles that curl or have fullness around the jaw are best avoided.

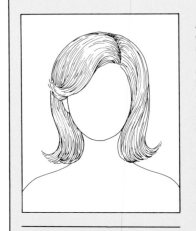

ROUND

A round face is often referred to as chubby or fat, though this is not necessarily the case. If you have a round face you should try to create as much height with your hair as possible, as this will give an illusion of length to the face and be sure to avoid too much hair on the face, as this can accentuate the roundness. If your hair type allows, tone down the roundness of your face with straight lines, and a flicked-out bob below the jawline, as the picture on the left illustrates. It is best to avoid bubbly perms, very heavy hairstyles and ringlets if you have a round face, unless you compensate for the curls by making sure that the hair is short at the cheek bones. Square and diagonal lines are usually the safest style to have as they are more flattering to a round face, because they give a more definite, stronger line to the whole head and face.

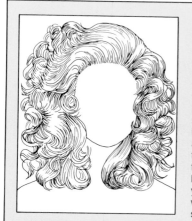

SQUARE

If your face shape is square, hard line haircuts - such as the geometric styles or long bobs with heavy straight fringes that have been fashionable since their introduction by Vidal Sassoon in the 1960s - should ideally be avoided as often as possible. You should aim to have a little added height, and make sure that you add width to the sides, between the eyebrows and lips to soften the squareness of your face. If the hair is long give a gentler line to your face by having it layered or wavy. As the picture to the left shows a long fringe can be swept up and back at the side and the result of this technique is to add width and curl to flatter the shape of the face. Notice that the curly hair at the sides of the head overlaps the face thus softening the cheek and jaw lines, and at the forehead and temples the hairline is curved around the face as much as possible, another technique that disguises the square shape.

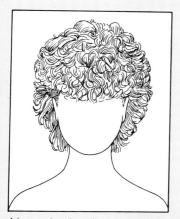

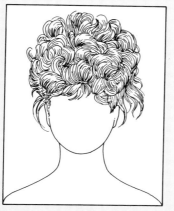

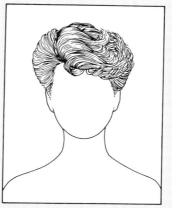

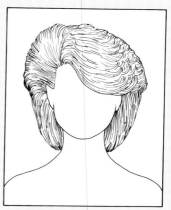

A layered curly style or permanent wavéd hair *can* look good on a round face. If you are determined to have curly hair, it will look best if care is taken to avoid a bubbly round look by ensuring that the hair is short at the cheek bones. In the illustration the length and colour of the hair behind the ears is used to sharpen the jawline.

In order to increase the height of the hair, and therefore the length of the face, layered hair is cut flat at the sides and shorter at the front. This gives lift from the forehead. The long hair at the back can be left down or pinned up for a more sophisticated look. To further enhance this style, fine wisps or fronds at the back and sides of the head and face will add a romantic feel to the look.

This is a very popular style. The line of the cut - from the short hair at the ears to the large volume of hair at the crown - gives the illusion of an oval face shape. The long waves that sweep across the forehead offer plenty of scope for highlighting and colour.

This style is neat and fashionable. The hair is blow dried away from the face at the sides. The heavy fringe falls asymmetrically over one eye and on the other side of the parting the hair has been swept up and back to give more height.

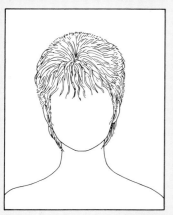

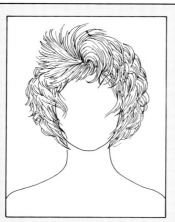

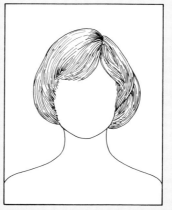

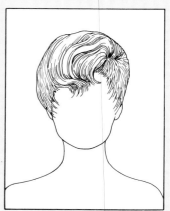

Square shaped faces may be able to carry off short sharp hairstyles, but only if this part of the hairstyle is made up for by having wisps of hair over the forehead. To break up the angular lines of the thick hair, as shown here, width is needed at the sides of the head.

This wispy bob-shaped cut, with tendrils that soften the forehead, cheeks and chin, creates a feminine look that will suit a variety of hair textures and age groups. The hair has been cut to varying lengths in sections around the head. Here the hair has been gelled, moussed and scrunch dried to give it extra texture, but the style can also be achieved by using heated rollers.

This face framing hair style is cut in a helmet-shaped style, which is slightly graduated at the cheeks and around the forehead at the parting to give a gentle look to the face. This style is suitable for straight, wavy or curly hair.

An asymmetrical style can work if the tips of the hair are left wispy and soft, to break up the square shape of the face.

Types of cut

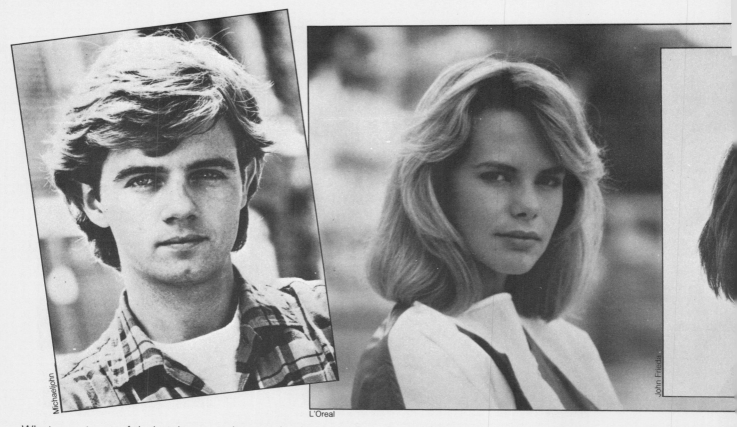

Michaeljohn

L'Oreal

John Frieda

Whatever type of hairstyle you choose, it should be something that you can maintain yourself so you can ensure that it stays in shape between visits to the hairdresser. Just how often you should have your hair cut depends on the style. As a general rule, the shorter the hair the more often you will need to have it trimmed. Short hair can quickly lose its shape, so, ideally, it should be cut every six weeks at the very least. Often, when people complain that their hair has been cut too short, the time left between visits has probably been too long and the stylist has had to cut off more than was asked for by the client, just to get back the basic shape.

Short hairstyles can be versatile, especially when cut with a fringe (bangs). One day the hair can be worn with the fringe covering the forehead, and the next it can be brushed back away from the face. If it is a changeable style you want, ask the hairdresser to advise you on the various possibilities.

Medium-to-long hair is also easily managed and, for most women, it is probably the most attractive length. It is preferable to really long hair for most women after their twenties. Of course, a compromise is to have hair that is shorter around the face and longer in the back.

The reason for cutting hair is not only to reduce its overall length or to remove damaged ends. The main objective is to give the hairstyle its basic shape.

The silhouette of the total head is of utmost importance. This is particularly true with curly hair. The intricacies of the style itself can easily get lost within a mass of curls, so the hairdresser must look at the overall shape to achieve a dramatic effect.

The haircut will depend to a large extent on the natural growth pattern and condition of the hair. Thick, coarse hair usually has enough body to hold a good short cut. Medium hair, if it is not naturally wavy, may be floppy and, like fine hair, may need a perm for extra body.

Part of your hairdresser's job will be to advise you on how to preserve your haircut. When you have been wearing your hair long for years, it may come as quite a shock that even a straight bob may need to be blow dried to look good. Long hair can be extremely deceptive. While it is long, it may look straight simply because there is a lot of weight pulling on it. Cut the hair and it may well be wavy. Also, when long hair is cut it may suddenly appear not to have the same amount of body simply because it has lost so much of its volume and it may well become fly-away.

When cutting the hair, the first thing the stylist will look for is the crown – or crowns, as some people have more than one – because the natural fall of the hair radiates from the crown of the head in all directions. The hairdresser will then establish where the natural parting

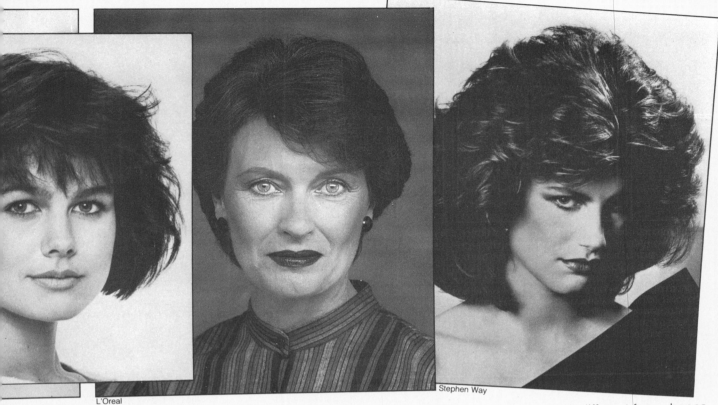

L'Oreal

Stephen Way

lies, as it is advisable to work with it, rather than against it. A false parting causes the hair to rise uncomfortably from the scalp, whereas with a true parting it will lie and radiate around the head naturally.

Cutting the hair while it is still wet gives better control, as wet hair is less slippery. Another advantage is that the outline of the head can be seen more clearly. And, of course, it is more hygienic for the stylist to handle freshly shampooed hair.

The bob

The classic bob is perhaps the oldest hairstyle known to man. Egyptian mummies are evidence that the style was in use thousands of years ago. Taking it right back to basics, the bob has the hair cut in a perfectly straight line from the nape to the chin. The variations on the theme are infinite. For example, the outline shape can be changed simply by tapering the cut so that it is either shorter at the back than at the front, or vice versa.

If you think that with a bob the hair is cut to one length you are in fact mistaken. The very fact that the head is round in shape means that the hair on the crown has to be a great deal longer than the hair in the nape – even when it looks exactly the same length in the end.

As a hairstyle the bob is very versatile, because it can

be worn at different lengths to suit different face shapes and varied with the amount of curve put into the very ends. Its simplicity means it never really goes out of fashion, yet it still has the classical lines of a very elegant hairstyle.

The layer cut

A layer cut is done in a completely different way. It involves taking sections of hair, holding them between the fingers at right angles to the scalp, and cutting these meshes at intervals of ½ to 1 inch (1.2 to 2.5 centimetres). Often a layer cut is combined with a bob. For instance, the outline shape can be a bob, but the interior of the hair is cut in long and short alternating layers to give texture and movement. A layer cut has to be done extremely well, especially when the hair is thick and straight, or it can end up looking very untidy. This is because the hair itself may lack natural movement, making it difficult for the stylist to get the hair to behave. Often the hairdresser will have to improvise to ensure that a particular wayward piece of hair can be turned under.

Hair is cut as an entity and each section of hair is cut in careful balance to the next. This is why you should never try and save on visits to the hairdresser by snipping off bits yourself. The danger is that you will destroy the balance of the whole haircut.

Basic cutting tools and techniques

The two main cutting tools used by hairdressers are scissors and razors. Dedicated followers of Vidal Sasson never choose a stylist who uses a razor on hair and, as a result, the razor as a haircutting instrument has somewhat gone out of favour. Originally, the reason for razor cutting was to thin or shape the hair to its desired weight. The hair had to be kept wet while the razor was being used. According to Sassoon and those who follow his styling methods, there are very few cases where hair needs to be thinned in the first place. Where it does, they think, scissors are preferable.

With scissors, the hairdresser can prune out just the amount necessary. With a razor, the danger is that it is easy to thin out more than required. Razor cutting is generally unsuitable for fine hair, but where there is plenty of hair, the technique can work. It can help achieve that spiky windblown look which, lifted with gels in any direction, can make for an exciting, tousled and swirling silhouette. Such spiky looks can create a version of the classic bob, often combining the blunt cut at the back with uneven layers that stand away from the top of the head to create lots of volume.

A hairdresser may or may not use a razor, but several pairs of scissors are indispensable. The scissors vary in blade length from around 4 inches (10 centimetres) for precision work such as fringes (bangs), to 5 inches (13 centimetres) or more for Afro hair. With strong, curly hair the longer blade is needed so that the hairdresser can place the hands further away from the hair as it is cut. This helps the hairdresser to see the overall shape while working on the the client's head of hair.

Most hairdressers, whether using scissors or razors, often use a straight-edged comb as a cutting guide. Sometimes thinning scissors are used rather than razors if the hair is thick or difficult to manage. Thinning scissors have one straight blade and one serrated cutting edge. They trim fewer hairs at one go than the usual hairdressing scissors, providing a more natural effect.

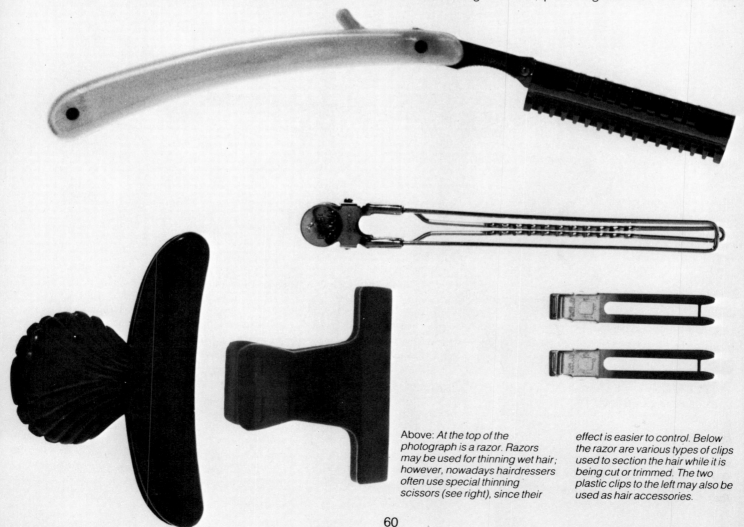

Above: *At the top of the photograph is a razor. Razors may be used for thinning wet hair; however, nowadays hairdressers often use special thinning scissors (see right), since their* *effect is easier to control. Below the razor are various types of clips used to section the hair while it is being cut or trimmed. The two plastic clips to the left may also be used as hair accessories.*

Clippers, once associated mostly with the 'short back and sides', are gaining favour again in both men's and women's hairdressing. The cutting head of hair clippers consists of two plates with serrated edges. One of the plates moves laterally over the other plate which is fixed. The hair is clipped at the point of contact between the serrations. Different models, either hand or electrically driven, are available. Most are adjustable so that they can cut almost as close as shaving, or they can leave the hair longer. Clippers must be used on dry hair.

The hairdresser will observe certain rules, whatever instrument used for thinning hair. It should never be thinned in the front hairline area, or on the top layers on either side of a parting or the top layer surrounding the crown. With naturally curly hair, it is usually best to have the hair blunt cut and kept one overall length that is thick at the ends rather than graduated. The reason is that, when the hair is thinned, it tends to swell and frizz. This can happen not only after washing, but even in a humid atmosphere. Conversely, if hair goes limp at the slightest sign of humidity in the air, accentuating its natural smoothness will cause the minimum fuss to keep in shape.

Techniques

It was Sassoon's idea to leave all the hair blunt cut, so that the ends are as thick as the roots, as hair is naturally. The technique of using scissors to remove carefully selected hairs or groups of hair is called pointing. This is often used for fringes. Pointing, involves using the points of the scissor and cutting the hair in alternating long and short lengths. The greater the contrast in alternating lengths, the stronger the effect.

Another cutting technique and one that can help make soft fine hair look good is called feathering. This involves individual sections of hair being cut in such a way so as to achieve a 'feathery' effect.

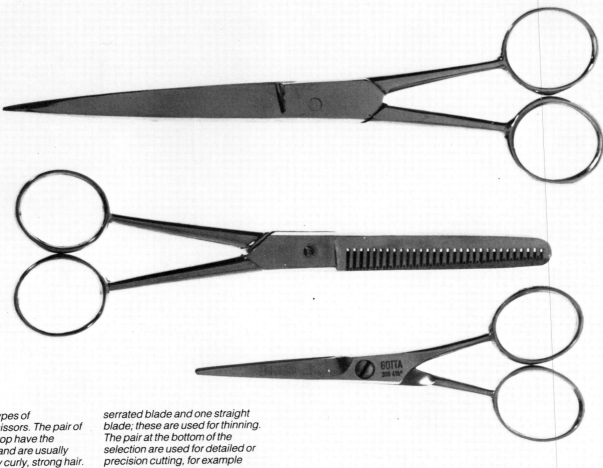

Above: *Three types of hairdressing scissors. The pair of scissors at the top have the longest blade, and are usually used to cut very curly, strong hair. The pair in the middle have one serrated blade and one straight blade; these are used for thinning. The pair at the bottom of the selection are used for detailed or precision cutting, for example cutting fringes.*

61

How to cut your hair

You cannot really include hair cutting among the do-it-yourself skills. It takes a special ability and artistry to provide a good shaping cut that falls into place – the right place – to enhance your hairstyle. But not everyone can get to the hairdressers regularly, either for economic or geographic reasons, so it is useful to know the basic principles of hair cutting in case you have to keep your hair in shape yourself or are called upon to look after the locks of your husband or boyfriend, your child or an elderly relative who is housebound. Also, it could be useful for maintaining a professional haircut, even for a short time, with a bit of trimming that follows the predetermined line.

Cutting bobs

For do-it-yourselfers, the easiest style to cope with is the bob, as it is cut to all one length. It uses a club (blunt) technique, a simple, straight-across cut that neatly evens out the tips and which is particularly suited to fine hair as it gives the appearance of more body by keeping weight at the ends.

No matter what type of hair you have, a bob cut can always be adapted to suit, because it is so versatile. Whatever the current hair fashions are, the bob will always remain a favourite, because it is easy to maintain. With regular trimming, it will hold its shape with a minimum of effort on your part and the hairdresser's. Its therefore extremely practical if you're short on both time and money. If you feel it lacks excitement, you can dramatize the looks with a colour rinse or streaks, tipping and frosting at the ends and with brightly-coloured accessories such as slides or ribbons to catch the hair back.

Layer cutting

With layer cutting, the hair is at different lengths on different parts of the head, to give a contoured shape or to tame an unruly mop. Layer cutting is often combined with tapering at the hair tips, which gives a softer and wispier look to the style. It is only suitable on hair that is short because on long hair the effect simply finishes up looking as if you have split ends.

Many of today's high-fashion effects can be achieved with layer-cutting. The technique involves the use of different hair lengths to achieve daring and dramatic effects. Layering is also useful if the hair is very coarse and curly, and helps to achieve a more controlled look. The 1980s layer cut styles often feature hair chopped very short on the crown so that it stands upright, with sleek, longer hair at the nape and temples.

Layer cutting, if done well, gives the illusion of movement, but it is definitely not ideal for every type of hair. If your hair is fine and straight, a soft perm or body

CUTTING A BOB

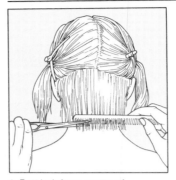

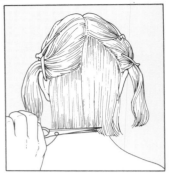

1. Part hair from centre of forehead to nape of neck. Clip all except bottom layer of hair into two bunches either side of head. Hold free hair with comb, pulling gently away from head, and cut.

2. Comb another section on right hand side of the head and cut to same level as previous section. Grip hair between the middle and index fingers and use comb as a guide to ensure the line is straight.

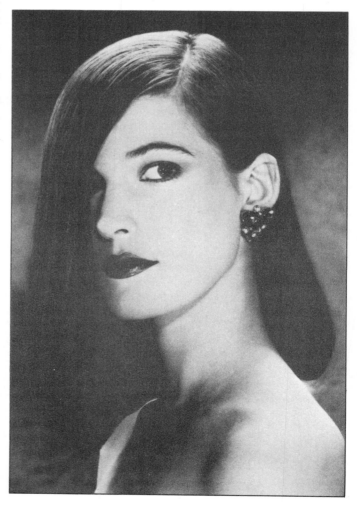

CUTTING A BOB

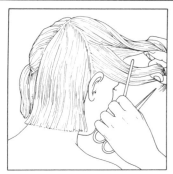

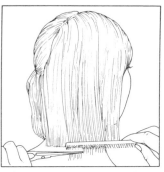

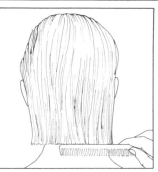

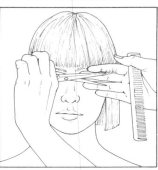

3. Take a further section from right hand side of the head and cut to the same level as the previous two sections, ensuring that hair is smooth and held taut.

4. Continue to comb out sections of hair on the right side of the head and repeat the cutting process, using the first cut section as a guide to the correct level of cut.

5. Cut hair on the left hand side of the head, matching the level of cut to previous sections. When you have finished, comb the hair into line and trim any stray ends.

6. If you want a fringe (bangs), cut this last of all. Cut from the centre of the forehead outwards and, when cutting, allow for fringe to dry shorter than when wet.

Warning: You will need to use sharp implements when cutting the hair. Make sure that care is taken to avoid injury and accidental damage to your hair

Variations on the bob – with side-parting, swept-back or full fringe. The versatility of the basic cut allows for different styling interpretations and all that remains constant is that the hair is cut to all one length, rather than layered, to give a smooth fall from roots to tips.

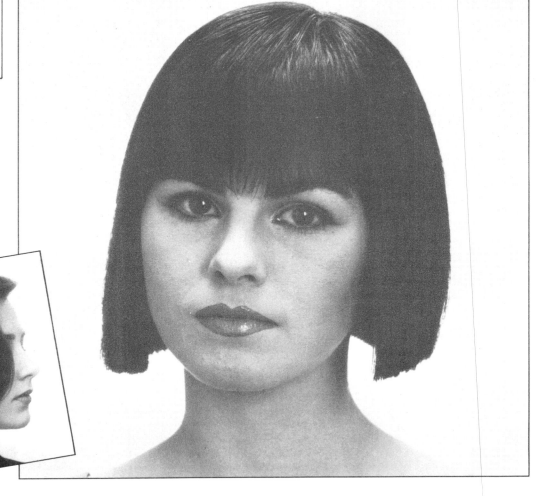

wave is usually an essential preliminary. Thick and slightly curly hair can respond well to layer cutting. Unless the cut is designed to hug the shape of the head, the upkeep can be troublesome and time-consuming, requiring the use of heated rollers or brushes and sometimes gels and mousses to maintain the shape and movement. Feathering is often used in layer cuts to give a flattering wispy effect to fringes, for example. It looks very pretty and feminine, but unless you intend to keep up the good work, you had better leave this type of style alone: wispy can soon become straggly!

Layer cuts need to be kept up regularly; if you leave your visits to the hairdresser too long, the chances are that the style will lose its shape and that it will become difficult to coax the hair the way you want it. The shorter layers often start to flop and split ends tend to be particularly noticeable.

Highlighting or bleaching the tips of layered hair can emphasize the silhouette and movement. If your hair needs a perm in order to make it suitable for layer-cutting, the haircut should be done as perfectly as possible before the perm is applied.

If you want to change back from a layer cut to a blunt cut bob, you will have to let it grow out gradually, at least until the top layer is long enough to hang to the nape of the neck. Once the hair falls to the nape it can be blunt cut and left to grow as long as you like.

Layering or tapering the hair is a difficult technique for

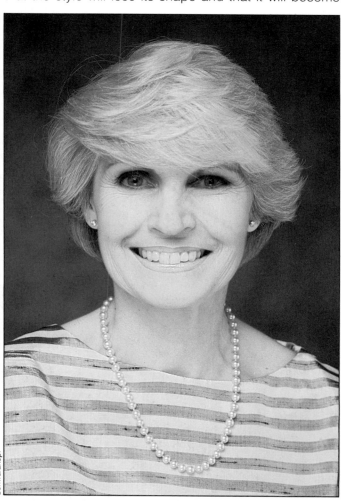

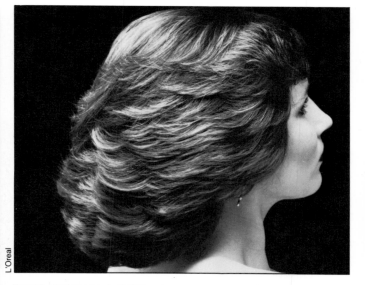

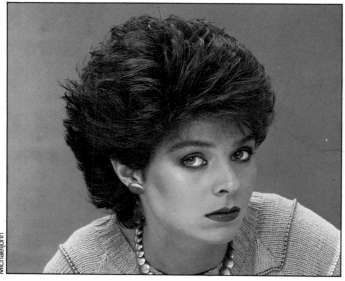

Layered hair is right for many styles to suit different ages and types. An older women (above) with a mass of thick hair can have a layer cut to control the hair's weight and volume. A young girl with fine hair can maintain a fuller look on long styling. Short hair (below right) achieves bounce and body.

Schwarzkopf

L'Oreal

Michaeljohn

you to achieve yourself, because there are always those odd sections at the back or the sides that you cannot easily reach or cannot see 'straight on' even with the help of triple mirrors. Far better on your own hair to stick to simple trimming.

Trimming layered hair

For this – as with any hair cutting – you need professional tools. It is no good attempting to tackle a cut with the kitchen scissors or dressmaking shears. Scissors need to have small, narrow blades that do not obscure the section of hair you are cutting and they need to be very, very sharp to give a good clean cut.

You will need to work on small sections of hair at a time, using the section you have just cut as a guideline for the next section. To maintain an even, balanced look, work from a central parting running from forehead to nape of the neck and work on damp hair which is easier to control and shows more accurately the natural line of the hair. Always cut the hair a little longer than you want it – that way you have room for manoeuvre and can make adjustments by taking off a little more length. Also the hair shortens a little as it goes from damp to dry – especially if there is quite a bit of natural curl – and a certain amount of length will be 'taken up' in the drying process.

With a rat tail comb, section off a slim section of hair about 2 inches (5 centimetres) wide and comb it at right angles to the scalp. Then hold the section of hair firmly between the index and middle fingers of your left hand (if you are right-handed) and slide them up the hair until they are just below the point you want to cut. Hold the scissors above your hand, parallel to the fingers that are holding the section of hair, and cut in one positive slicing movement, rather than snipping at the hair. Comb hair through and then take up the next strand, overlapping it with some of the cut strand to guide you to the exact level you should make the second cut. Work from ear to ear across the top of the head to complete the front sections and then back again from ear to ear across the back of the head for the back sections. Keep combing to check for length and evenness, especially on the front sections at each side of the head where just the slightest fraction of a difference in length would cause a lopsided look.

Hold the hair at right angles to the head for the straightest cutting effect and never at an oblique or shallow angle. When you have finished cutting, however, comb the hair straight down, pressing the tips close to the sides of your face and neck, and trim the very ends into a uniform straight line.

When it comes to cutting a fringe (bangs), special care must be taken to follow the curve of the forehead to keep the line straight above the eyebrows. Press the hair down firmly or tape it into position with setting tape and cut from the centre, working towards one side and then towards the other. Remember that the hair, once dry, will lift up, so cut at least ½ inch (1.2 centimetres) below the level you want to wear your fringe (bangs).

Stick to fairly simple trimming and do not be tempted to try anything too ambitious. Only when you feel fairly confident about handling the scissors and have had practice with a basic club-cutting (blunt cutting) technique, either on your own or on others' hair, should you attempt tapering or thinning.

TRIMMING LAYERED HAIR

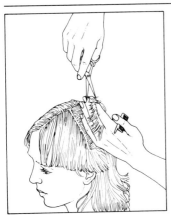 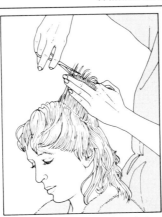 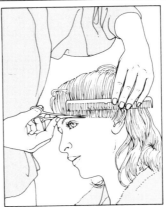 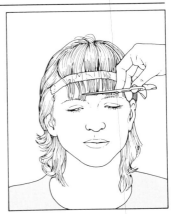

1. Section from centre forehead to nape of neck take 2 inch (5 centimetre) sections, in turn, from centre parting to ear.

2. Holding hair out at 90° angle to head, slide fingers up the section of hair until you reach required length, cut along the straight line made by your fingers.

3. When you have finished cutting all the sections in this way, comb the hair straight down, press the tips close to the sides of the face and neck, and snip off any straggly bits of hair.

4. Press hair down across forehead and tape it into position, and work from the centre of the forehead out to the side, first one side then the other. Don't cut off too much to start with.

Cutting curly, layered hair

The advantage of cutting curly hair is that the ends do not have to be so precisely cut because an uneven line is not going to show up among a mass of curls and movement. However, the disadvantage is that it is difficult to comb into the correct lines to follow while cutting, so it is hard to maintain a shape for the style you want.

Cutting can be used as a method for controlling an over-curly head of hair, simply by creating a shape in exactly the same way that straight hair is cut in exact lines. With curly hair the cut can create a contoured look and hold the hair close to the head. You can see the variety of shapes that can be achieved if you look at Afro hairstyles, where the hair can be cut into a square shape on top of the head or into a round halo effect.

How much curly hair depends on a superb cut was demonstrated by Vidal Sassoon in 1967 when he created the 'Greek Goddess' look and proved that by using his precision-cutting technique hair could be permed and left to dry naturally. It was the first of the successful wash-and-dry styles that revolutionized hairdressing.

Generally speaking, curly hair looks better with a short to medium length, which is easier to handle than long hair that can easily look unruly unless perfectly groomed all the time. Because you want to control the ends of the curls to make them turn in on themselves, tapering or feather cutting is a better technique than club cutting (blunt cutting).

Curly hair is better cut while just damp rather than really wet so the true formation of the curl can be seen and the cutting can be adjusted accordingly.

If you have curly hair and want to wear it long, then it is better to keep it all one length and thick at the ends rather than graduated. This gives a little weight that will pull the hair into wavy rather than curly movement.

The type of style you choose will determine how often you need a haircut and whether your hair is straight or curly. Hair grows at a rate of approximately ½ inch (1.2 centimetres) a month, and obviously a ½ inch on a very short style will be more noticeable than it will on a head of long hair. So with short hair you need more regular visits to the hairdresser or more frequent trimming at home. Short and medium hair that has been cut to all one length, in a style such as the classic bob, will show up any variation of length and unevenness far more noticeably than a layer cut will and is likely to need more frequent trimming to keep its line and shape.

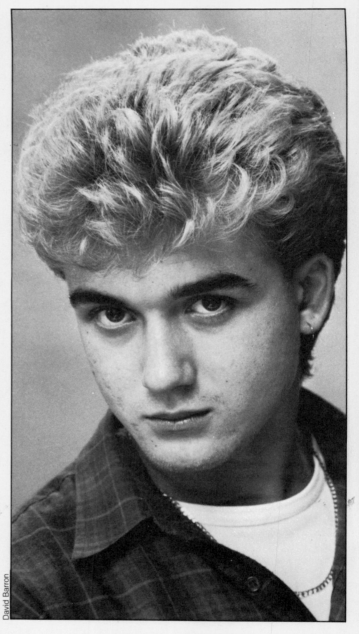

David Barron

Tapering hair

To taper hair, instead of cutting square across the ends, you cut at a slant, and the sharper the angle the scissors make with the hair, the greater the tapering effect. Each hair in the section that has been cut will vary in length so the very tip of the section is thinner than the rest of it. It makes the ends look wispier and gives a feathery effect.

One disadvantage of the tapering technique is that it increases the risk of split ends, especially on hair that is dry or out-of-condition. So if curly hair would benefit from club (blunt) cutting to strengthen the ends, a tapering effect can be achieved with layer cutting, where the hair sections are in fact club (blunt) cut but in layers of different length up the head, with the shortest lengths at the top and crown, graduating down to longer sections at the back and sides.

Cutting children's hair

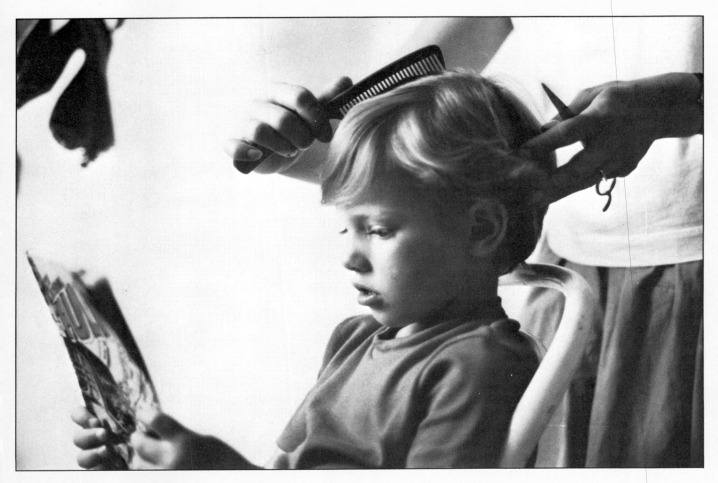

Most mothers cut their children's hair believing it to be extravagant to take a young child to a hairdressing salon. But, in fact, you are never too young to have your hair shaped in a good style, and it pays once in a while to have a good professional cut for your child that you can keep in trim yourself by following the line set by the hairdresser. There is one school of thought that says you should not cut baby curls because it will cause the hair to grow straight. But, in fact, baby curl is often only a temporary stage of hair growth and it will disappear anyway, so there is little point in hanging on to it.

Also, babies' hair often tends to get knotted at the back of the head where they lie on it, so it is worth getting it cut into shape to prevent this kind of tangling problem that is prevalent with very fine hair.

The hair will gradually thicken as your baby grows into a child, but, during the early years of a child's life, the hair is usually very fine and fly-away, with a tendency to dryness, so it needs careful handling. Also, because few children seem to have the ability to sit still for more than a few minutes at a time, trying to cut the hair of a natural fidget can be troublesome for a mother, whereas a professional hairdresser is used to handling 'difficult' clients and will take cutting a child's hair in his or her stride. Moving around and tantrums will be smartly dealt with!

If you do trim your child's hair at home, make sure he or she is at the right level for you, so you do not have to bend or stoop at an unnatural angle. Cut hair while damp for more control, and, as fine hair tends to dry quickly, it is worth having a waterspray bottle to dampen the hair during the cutting process.

Use club-cutting (blunt cutting) techniques that give hair a bit of weight at the end and add an impression of fullness to fine hair. Keep the style simple and easy to maintain on a day-to-day basis – you can always dress up a little girl's hair with ribbons and bows for partytime – and keep fringes (bangs) and front hair short enough to avoid the eyes.

Encourage children to take an interest in their hair from an early age and, it is hoped, they will be interested in hair care for the rest of their lives. Also, it helps set them on the right road for taking a pride in their appearance generally.

Beards and moustaches

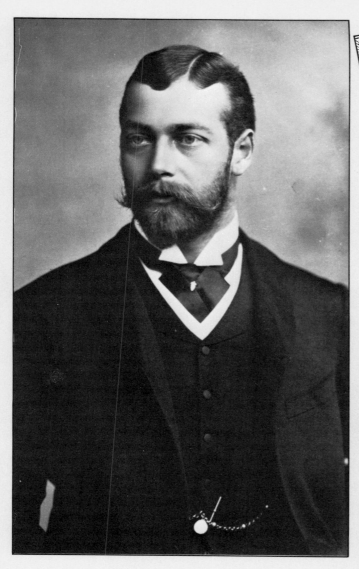

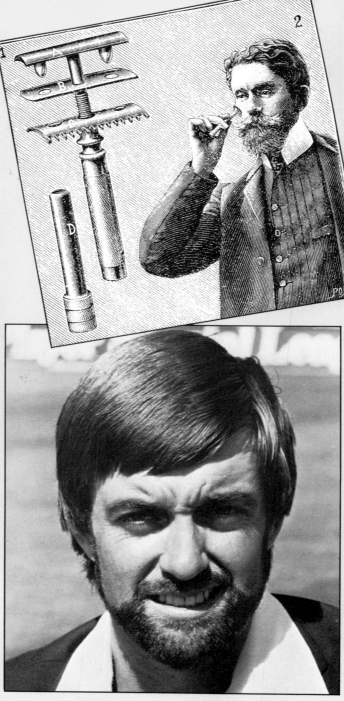

Beards have gone in and out of fashion almost as frequently as women's hairstyles. In ancient civilizations, beards were a traditional part of the male fashion. Even until quite recently, the Chinese considered a long beard to be a wonderful adornment. As for the Turks, they thought it more infamous to have their beard shaved than to be publicly whipped.

Sometimes a beard is just impractical, as many a historical precedent has shown. Alexander the Great ordered his troops to shave in order to deprive the enemy of a convenient grip to help them decapitate their opponents in battle. Beards were worn by the Saxons in England but short hairstyles and beardless faces were the order of the day after the Norman Conquest. During the reign of Elizabeth I, the growth of beards was

The beard has had a fascinating history and was popular in the nineteenth century, approved of by the Prince of Wales. George V (above left) followed on the Royal tradition with a neatly trimmed set of whiskers. Beards became less fashionable, with the invention of *the safety razor. Gillette (top right)patented the safety razor circa 1905 and shaving became easier. Beards have gained in popularity with neatly trimmed styles (below right) most frequently favoured.*

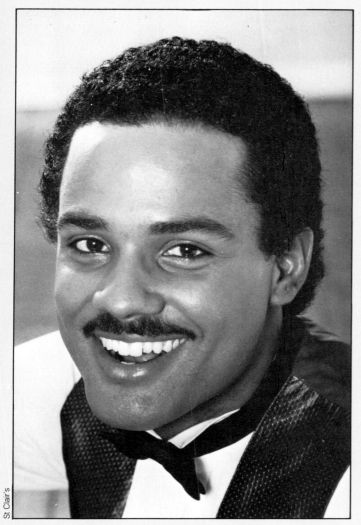

St Clair's

Above: *Moustaches create a good image but need shaping to suit face.*

a shorter man. A beard can make immature features look more striking. A moustache can help compensate for sunken cheekbones, whereas a beard can hide a receding chin. On the other hand, if the chin is too prominent, a beard can draw attention to it, while a moustache can help to make it less noticeable. Never wear a beard or moustache when you have a low forehead.

Beards

A beard must not only look good, it must also feel good. It should be soft to the touch, even if the hair is strong and curly. The secret could be the way the beard is trimmed. Beards should be trimmed with scissors rather than a razor or clippers. Trimmed with very sharp scissors, the hair is cut at a slanting angle and this makes it feel smooth and soft. The clipper and razor give a blunt edge to the hair which creates an unpleasant, stubbly feeling. If the beard hair is rather difficult to control, it is a good idea to use both shampoo and conditioner. This can also help prevent dryness of the skin underneath.

It can be quite tricky to trim the beard at the sides of the face and, when a beard has grown for the first time, it may be advisable to enlist the help of a barber or friend. The beard is always most easily cut when it is damp, after shampooing and conditioning.

Thoroughly comb the beard first to remove any tangles. A straight-edged comb can be used as a cutting guide. It should be placed teeth upwards against the hair, so that the hair sticks through the teeth and the beard can be trimmed away. Take it slowly and do a little at a time, being particularly careful around the lip area which is always rather delicate.

It is definitely not a good idea to grow a beard just to save time shaving. For a beard to look good, it will need a lot of time spent on it; shampooing, trimming and combing can take just as long, if not longer, as a morning shave.

Moustaches

There was something of a compromise during and after World War I, when most men shaved, but full moustaches were in favour at the same time. A beard and a moustache can make a man look more masculine, as well as helping to camouflage imperfections.

Older men should be particularly careful not to sport a drooping moustache. The moustache could have the effect of making the features look as though they are sagging. This is the last thing you will want, particularly when the years are creeping up, and if you are not careful you could easily be making yourself look older than you are.

regulated by statute. An order was imposed that no man of the Queen's household should wear a beard above a fortnight's growth. If he did, he would risk the penalty of a fine, loss of commons and, finally, expulsion.

The hair and beard needed much dressing, and, in the sixteenth and seventeenth centuries, it was common practice to dye the beard, both to fit in with fashion and also to disguise age.

As do-it-yourself shaving became much easier after the safety razor was invented, the clean-shaven look has won the day for most men in this century.

Like a hairstyle, the beard or moustache should never be considered in isolation. Height, hairstyle, facial features – all have to be taken into account. If you are tall, it would suit you better to wear a fuller beard than it would

At the hairdresser

One thing to remember when you visit your hairdresser is that there is a lot of competition in this business; if you are not satisfied you can always try your luck elsewhere. On the other hand, it is important that you give the hairdresser a chance by not making impossible demands. Instead, talk over the possibilities and find out exactly what you can or cannot expect before you decide on a new style. Most hairdressers are happy to fit in with your ideas, provided these are practical. If the stylist quizzes you about your life-style and about the type of clothes you normally wear, he or she is not being nosy for the sake of it. You will need to communicate with the hairdresser as much as he or she needs to with you, so that your hairstyle can be 'tailor-made' and the result achieved will please you both.

Your own hair type plays an important part in dictating the style. This means that you should not have too fixed an idea in your head of what you want – and also that you should try to learn about the limitations your hair can impose. Perming or straightening can correct some problems when hair is either excessively wavy or very straight. A blunt cut that is not much longer than the chin may be best if the hair is fine and thin, whereas, if the hair is coarse, it may need to have a slightly longer cut.

By all means, show the hairdresser some pictures of hairstyles you like. There is nothing worse for the stylist than working without any knowledge of whether a client really wants the style he or she is planning. If your ideas will not work, ask the hairdresser to explain and, assuming you have faith in his or her abilities, do not go against professional advice. If you do not agree with the stylist's advice, it can only mean that this hairdresser is not for you and you will know for the next time. It may mean switching to a completely new salon or asking a different stylist in your existing salon to do your hair.

Finding a new hairdresser

Finding a new hairdresser is not unlike finding another dentist. How do you know you have picked the right one? One advantage for a client in attending a particular hairdresser is that every head styled is an advertisement – or not as the case may be – for the salon.

If you have a friend or colleague whose hairstyle you particularly like, that is as good a recommendation as any. Ring the salon and, if you do not want to take chances, ask if they are prepared to give you a consultation first. Many do so free of charge. Some salons also hold special client evenings when you have an opportunity to see a whole range of styles being created. The hairdressing business is known as a 'service industry'; it is a service that you pay for – and no one in the salon, from the owner down to the receptionist and assistant stylist, should ever forget this.

Top hairdressers are artists as well as craftsmen. You may be suprised to find that the new salon practies a totally different cutting technique from the one you were previously used to. If this is the case, remember that, while your hair is being done, you are in no position to argue. It is the final result that matters. You wouldn't argue for example, with your dentist about his technique of filling your teeth. It may be a week or more before you finally know whether your style works, and if you are not satisfied, by all means go back and tell your hairdresser. Even then, be reasonable: it may take more than one cut before the stylist really gets to know you and your hair. As you are a walking advertisement of the stylist's skills, he or she will do everything to try to satisfy your needs.

Once you have established a good relationship with the stylist, you should have no problems. When you feel you have cause for complaint, then try to settle matters as quietly and as amicably as possible. Most good salons will try to appease you somehow even if that means just giving you advice on caring for the style at home. It may take some while to get used to a short haircut, but if it is a style you chose in the first place, it will be your responsibility and not the salon's. With really top hairdressing salons, technical errors on the part of the staff are rare: most will have had years of training and experience.

Time and money

Limited funds or lack of time can be further limitations. Few people these days can go for a hair cut more often than about every five to six weeks. This means that the hair has to keep in shape between visits; it may also have to be very adaptable, so that you can change it once in a while. If you are constantly in a hurry, this may mean a style than can be towel-dried, combed and left to dry naturally. This is no problem if the hair has the right texture: if it is thick and bouncy. Unfortunately, fine, limp hair usually needs blow drying to give it a little more volume; the hairdresser can show you how this is done.

Accidents

If, very occasionally, a client is injured accidentally, there is, of course, the possibility of claiming for personal injury. It could happen that a perming lotion causes an allergic reaction, even after all the correct test procedures have been carried out on a small area on the scalp. In such a case, it is important that you go to a doctor immediately, as you will need a medical report to back up any personal injury claim. In all cases, have a word first with the owner or manager who will generally be grateful for an opportunity to set matters right so you will not need to take things further.

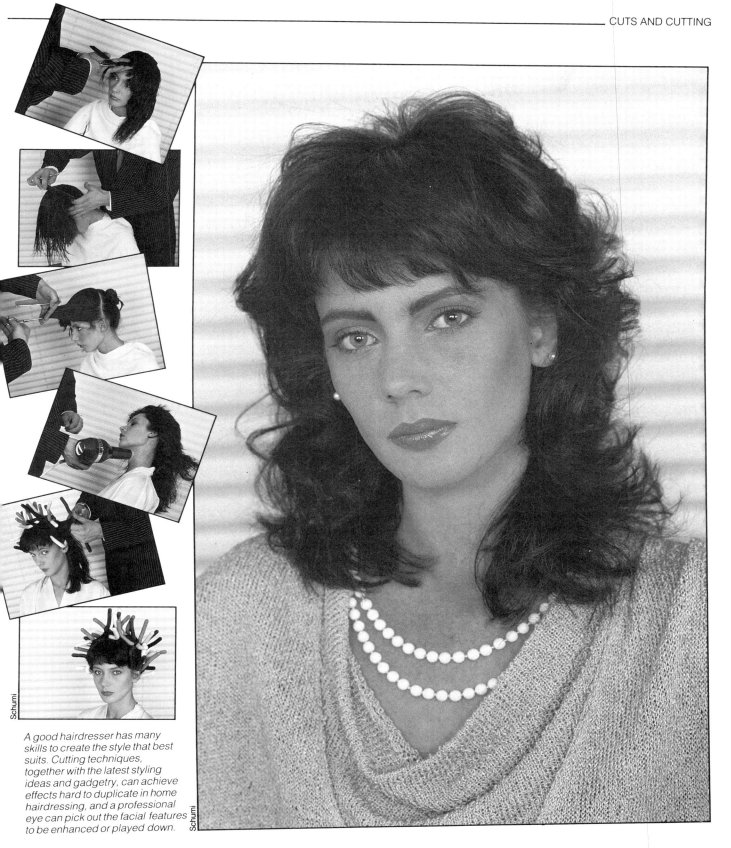

A good hairdresser has many skills to create the style that best suits. Cutting techniques, together with the latest styling ideas and gadgetry, can achieve effects hard to duplicate in home hairdressing, and a professional eye can pick out the facial features to be enhanced or played down.

Schumi

6
Colouring your hair

Ice cool blond, flaming redhead or sultry brunette – these are catchphrases that give some indication of the positive attitude we have towards hair colour. They indicate, too, that we tend to think of only three basic hair colourings – blond, red and brunette – but, of course, there are so many different shades in these three colours that the range is infinite.

Natural hair colour

The natural colour of hair is determined by the amount and type of melanin present in the centre of the hair shaft. Tiny melanin cells containing mixtures of brown, black, red and yellow pigment lodge in the cortex – or central layer – of each hair to provide the tone and intensity of hair colour. The outside of the hair shaft, the cuticle, is transparent, allowing the colour to shine through.

What colour your hair is depends on the combination of the melanin pigment. If it is mainly black and brown your hair will be dark brunette, while a predominance of red and yellow cells gives a much lighter shade of hair. Where red pigment is present in any great quantity, the hair will take on a warm tone. When mixed with black and brown, for instance, the red will produce an auburn shade, and mixed with yellow pigment it will create a strawberry-blond effect.

When the melanin cells in the cortex stop producing colour the hair becomes white as colourless air bubbles replace the pigment in the hair shaft. There is no such colour as grey in the hair. What is referred to as 'grey' hair is actually a mixture of white and naturally coloured hair that gives an overall effect of grey. Greying hair is part of the ageing process and occurs gradually over a period of several years as the melanin cells produce less and less pigment, so the effect is a slow fading of hair colour rather than a sudden dramatic colour loss.

Colour loss

If hair goes white at an early age it is usually a question of heredity and the colour loss occurs over a much shorter period. White hair often grows in a coarser texture than coloured hair, so youngsters who are grey frequently tend to have a luxuriant head of hair.

Another factor that can contribute to a sudden loss of hair colour is damage to the scalp, such as receiving a blow to the head. Usually white hair will be confined to the patch of scalp where the damage was inflicted, leaving a clearly defined white streak through the hair. Similarly, it is often the case with men that greying starts at the temples.

For many people the onset of greying is a worry because it is identified with ageing. It can cause psychological problems, especially if the greying starts considerably in advance of one's contemporaries. If there is an in-built fear of growing older, the visible signs will certainly not be welcomed and will need to be disguised. It is for this reason that many people – and that includes men as well as women – start using hair dye.

Using hair dyes and colourants

Apart from combatting the tell-tale signs of ageing, the use of a hair dye, in the form of a rinse or tint, is a way of conforming and blending in with the people around you. Hair that is different – whether by style or colour – is a very positive way of standing out in a crowd and, except for a minority who are exhibitionists, people do not generally like to be different. So Latins, with their dark colouring, might be superficially attracted to the idea of the Nordic blond as a symbol of beauty, and the fair-haired races may appreciate the dramatic possibilities of dark hair colouring; but it is usually attraction to the opposite colouring to oneself rather than the real wish to assume a completely different head of hair.

The use of hair dyes and colourings is usually, then, to enhance and improve on the natural, or to disguise changes that are taking place, rather than to make drastic alterations. The exceptions to this are cases where high, flamboyant colour is used – mainly by the young – to create striking, high-fashion looks. It is, for example, possible to have 1,000 different colours in your hair at the same time!

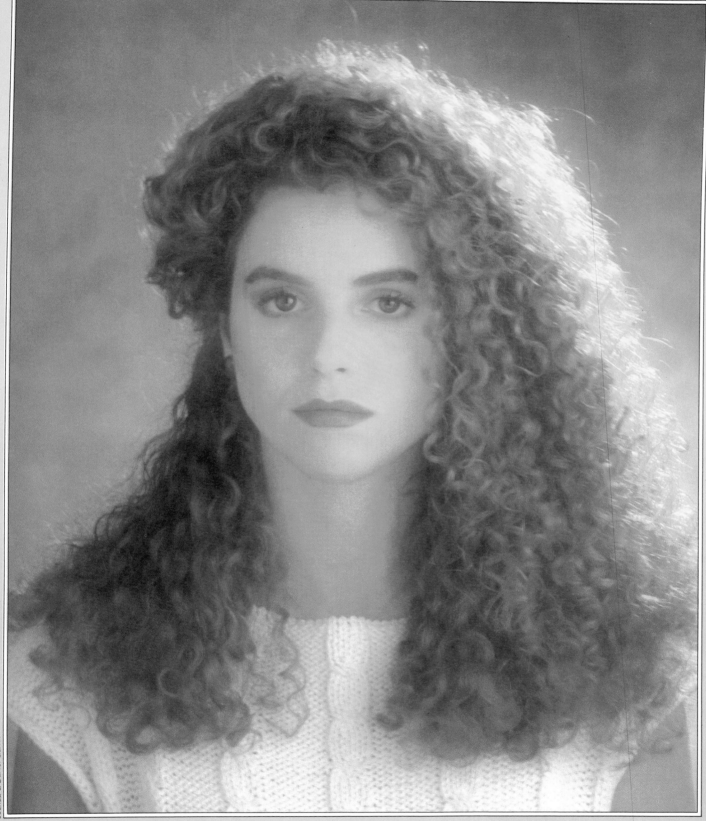

Types of colourant

To change the natural colour of your hair you need to rinse, tint or bleach it. A rinse lightly coats the outer layer – the cuticle – of the hair shaft with a colouring element. A tint penetrates the middle layer – the cortex – to combine with the natural colour contained there, and a bleach, depending on its strength, acts to remove part or all of the natural colour from the cortex.

The type of colourant you use will depend on whether you want just the subtlest hint of a tint, a dramatic change of colour or something between the two. It will also depend on the hair's own natural colour, its texture and what kind of condition it is in.

Health

In all cases it must be remembered that colour reduction may affect the condition of the hair, drying it out and

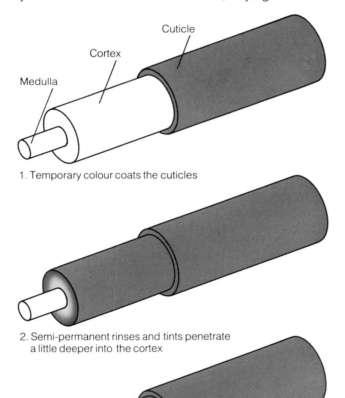

1. Temporary colour coats the cuticles

2. Semi-permanent rinses and tints penetrate a little deeper into the cortex

3. Permanent tints colour through the cortex to the medulla

making it sensitive not only to re-tinting but to permanent waving because of porous tips and general dryness. So always re-condition the hair thoroughly after any colour reduction treatment and make sure the hair is looking and feeling good before using any other chemical process on it, or you may further damage your hair.

Temporary colourant

The mildest form of hair colouring is a temporary colourant, a weak dye that stains the outer surface of each hair, turning its natural colour a shade or two deeper or adding a richness of tone that emphasizes natural – or bleached-in – highlights. It is also useful for toning down brassy effects of bleached hair and for enhancing grey and white hair, especially where yellowing or weathering effects have caused patchiness of colour.

The oldest type of temporary colour is the rinse, usually in powder form but sometimes in liquid or cream form, that needs to be dissolved or diluted in hot water. It is applied to hair that has been shampooed, thoroughly rinsed and towel-dried, and simply combed through to ensure even distribution. The hair is then left to dry naturally or with the help of a hair dryer.

The colour effect depends very much on the strength of the rinse you use and how much deeper than your natural hair colour the chosen shade is. For instance, a dark chestnut rinse will give an appreciable change of shade on light brown hair, whereas a light brown rinse will be scarcely noticeable when applied to dark chestnut hair. But even if you have made a mistake with your colour choice and you have added a too dark effect, there is no need to worry unduly, because temporary rinses can be easily removed by shampooing.

Temporary colourants are generally regarded as safe, so a skin test is not necessary. They don't contain the strong ingredients required to make chemical changes to the hair that are found in permanent dyes. In fact, many temporary colourants are made with food-stuff colourings which naturally enough are non-toxic.

For successful results you must take care to ensure you apply the rinse evenly and all through the hair. A hurried and slapdash application can all too easily end in streaky or patchy results.

More recent forms of temporary colour are dual-purpose. They come incorporated into shampoos or combined with setting lotion.

The shampoos have the advantage of cleaning and slightly colouring at the same time. Use half the application in the normal way to get rid of grease and dirt, rinse hair thoroughly and then re-shampoo, leaving the lather on the hair for five minutes or so before rinsing again. This gives the colour a chance to penetrate the hair's cuticles.

The coloured setting lotions are applied to towel-dried hair immediately after shampooing. The dyes are dissolved in resin and plastic bases that fix colour on to the hair as well as providing a fixative that helps hold a hairstyle in place. This base has to provide a light coating of colour on the hair shaft that will be reasonably rainproof, yet still removable with an ordinary thorough shampooing.

Other forms of temporary colouring are the spray-on, paint-on and puff-on, which are applied to hair that has been styled, to add sparkle or streaks of contrasting colour. These are the fun temporaries, mainly developed for parties. Many of them add glitter or have a metallic gold, silver, copper or bronze sheen, others come in bright shades of blue, yellow or red for dramatic highlights. Apart from their decorative use they can be helpful in disguising faults by blocking out the odd patch of grey or by enhancing a grey streak.

Because they are applied to hair that is dry, they don't have staining properties and so can be brushed out easily. Take care, for although they don't stain the hair, they can stain fabrics, so apply carefully and avoid the risk of colouring collars and necklines, too.

CHECKLIST FOR USING TEMPORARY COLOUR	
○ Before applying rinse, thoroughly blot-dry hair with a towel to remove surplus moisture that would otherwise dilute the rinse.	○ Don't mix rinses to form new shades. Some colours do not mix safely together and results can be unpredictable.
○ Always follow directions on bottle or tube concerning recommended dilution and don't be tempted to lessen dilution for stronger results.	○ Use hot water when mixing rinse. The warmth helps open the cuticles of the hair, allowing the rinse to penetrate below the surface.

Semi-permanent colourant

Midway between the temporary rinse and the permanent tint, comes the semi-permanent tint, which is a colouring compromise. It is formulated to penetrate a little way into the hair shaft and give a greater density of colour than the temporaries and it will last through approximately six shampoos. As the colour gradually fades with each successive shampooing there is no strong demarcation line between the tinted hair and the natural regrowth, so there is no need for the constant root retouching treatments necessary with permanent tints.

It also differs from permanent tints in that no activator – such as hydrogen peroxide – is needed so there is no mixing of two ingredients before application. Semi-permanent tints mostly come in shampoo form, which is

easy to apply, or in a gel or cream form that is applied with a sponge or a brush. They penetrate halfway into the hair shaft and effectively colour the hair within minutes of application. The longer a semi-permanent is left on, the stronger the shade will be. But don't leave it on for longer than the recommended time – or you might get a too-permanent result!

The main use of a semi-permanent colourant is to disguise the first signs of grey hair or to darken and intensify the natural colour of your hair. They will effectively blend in an even sprinkling of white hairs, although they can't disguise a concentrated patch of white. They work well for toning down brassy shades and will give an effective depth of colour to the natural hair shade.

For instance, brunette hair can be made to look darker and richer with a blue-black shade of semi-permanent; and ash-toned tints help even out those pepper-and-salt effects that often signal the onset of greying, but they can't give a drastic change of colour. This is because they don't rely on a chemical reaction for their results, so it is not necessary to have a skin test before using a semi-permanent tint.

Permanent colourant

For a definite change of hair colour that does not shampoo out you need a permanent tint. It completely penetrates the hair shaft, adds a greater depth of colour than a semi-permanent, and effectively covers hair with a large percentage of white, to give an even overall colour.

Most permanent colourants contain a chemical known as 'para', which is short for paraphenylenediamine or paratoluenediamine aniline derivative dye. There are exceptions, including a few dyes made from vegetable sources or metal-based colourants, mainly termed colour restorers, but para is the most widely used.

It is a chemical that can cause allergy problems for some people, so it is always wise to test your skin's tolerance to the dye before you start tinting, especially if you are colouring your hair for the first time or if you know you suffer from a sensitive skin.

The permanent effect of these tints is achieved with a colour activator, usually a peroxide or oxidant, which means a product made up of two elements – either two liquids or a powder and a liquid – which have to be mixed together before use. The activator creates a reaction that releases and then traps colour molecules deep within the hair shaft. This colour cannot be washed out which means you have to wait until the hair grows out to get rid of the colour. If you are happy to keep the colour indefinitely, it means, of course, that you are going to have to tint the new hair growth every four to five weeks as a band of natural colour begins to show up at the roots.

A major advantage of permanent tints is that they can create colour results lighter than your own natural shade because the peroxide or oxidant activator will bleach out colour from the hair. This gives a great scope for colour choice that can vary several degrees lighter or darker than your own colouring. The major disadvantage is the regular root retouching. However, as many products come packed in an applicator bottle with a long nozzle, it is easy to apply tint along the partings to the new growth first and allow time for the tint to work before combing or brushing it through the rest of the hair. This method of application helps prevent colour build-up along the lengths of hair that have been previously treated.

CHECKLIST FOR USING PERMANENT TINT

Here are some simple rules to ensure success in choosing and using a permanent tint:

O Ideally, choose a shade just a little lighter than your natural hair colour.

O If you are in your late forties or over, choose a light, natural-looking colour and avoid dark colours that give an ageing 'solid' look.

O If you have quite a lot of white in your hair, avoid using a reddish shade of colourant.

O If the hair is in poor condition, do not tint. Concentrate on improving the state of the hair first.

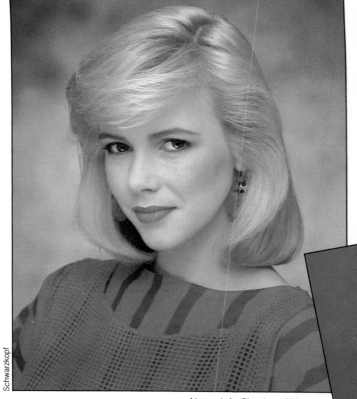

Schwarzkopf

Above left: Shades of blonde can be subtle and muted, or bold and brassy, as required.

The rich auburn red tones of this style incorporate lighter, brighter colour tones to emphasize the cut and curl of the hair shape.

Clipso

Bleaching

The reverse of colouring the hair is bleaching, a process that takes colour out of the hair – but the effect is still a permanent colour change that lasts until the treated hair grows out. Bleaches can range from a mild brightener that merely lifts the hair a shade or two, to the stronger products that strip out the natural colour entirely. Different types of bleach products are used to produce these varying results and, apart from the strength of the bleach, how much colour you take out of the hair depends on its natural shade, condition and texture and how long the bleaching product is left on the hair.

Bleach destroys the colour pigments in the hair, breaking down the black and brown ones first and then the red and yellow ones that are most resistant. On very dark or particularly warm-toned hair, bleaching does not remove all the colour – the hair would break up before that could happen – so a significant amount of the red and yellow pigments will remain. That is why poorly bleached hair so often ends up with a brassy or orange tinge.

The most powerful bleach mixes powder with high volume peroxide to give a paste that will strip colour from the hair until you are left with a platinum blond effect. Lower strength peroxide provides lesser effects, as do oil

Warning: Bleaching preparations contain active chemicals that can be dangerous if used incorrectly. If in doubt, take professional advice.

and cream-based bleaches mixed with peroxide compounds. They are ideal for creating the milder lightening effects, such as giving a lift to faded fair colouring, bringing out the natural highlights in mousey and mid-brown hair or enhancing the warm tones in dark and auburn hair.

Bleaching can be used to achieve a lot of different effects. Often it needs to be coupled with a colouring or toning process for maximum attraction. Where a strong lightening process or complex colouring work is needed, the treatment is best left to the hairdresser, whose professional expertise can judge just how much your hair can take. Careless use of too strong bleach or over-processing can dry out the hair, leaving it either brittle and prone to break or split-ended and looking like straw.

And, like permanent hair colouring, regular root

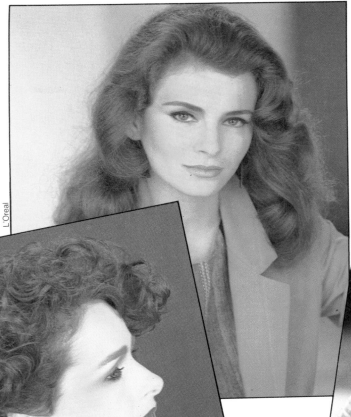

L'Oreal

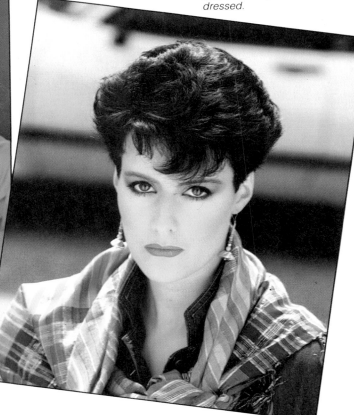

Kevin Michael

There are as many shades of brown and brunette as there are types and styles of hair. Colourants will enhance or disguise the hair's natural tone and create various effects to suit a particular style. The subtle red tones of the style on the left perfectly match the model's air of casual sophistication and simply dressed hair, while the rich raven colouring of the style below adds dramatic emphasis to a hairdo that is carefully contrived, cut and dressed.

retouching treatments are necessary to keep up the colour.

Patch and strand tests

When someone complains that a hair product didn't work or they did not get the result they had expected, it is usually because they did not read the instructions carefully or they cut corners to save time – very dangerous risks to take when colouring your hair.

To ensure you avoid problems and get the best results you need to spend a little time testing the product you intend to use. Check first to see what sort of colour effect the product will produce on your hair and check also that the product is safe to use on your skin.

Patch test for skin allergy. Some people are allergic to strawberries or shellfish; you might be allergic to a particular dye compound in a permanent tint. Simply dab cotton wool soaked in colourant behind your ear, or on the inside of the arm at the wrist or elbow. Allow tint to dry, then cover with a plaster and leave for 24 hours. If any irritation develops, you and the tint are incompatible. If there is no reaction you can go ahead and tint.

Strand test for colour result. Colour charts that come with the product are only a guide, not an exact prediction of the final result. Two heads of hair may look alike but actually vary enormously in basic red or yellow content, so check for effect on a strand of your own hair before colouring or bleaching. If part of your hair is grey, bleached, permed or already tinted, take a strand from that section as well as from the back of the head. Apply colourant according to instructions on the pack.

Using natural dyes

Herbal aids to health and beauty are as old as the hills, yet at the same time as new as today's scientific research and formulation. Plant extracts, taken from leaf, flower, root, seed or bark, in the form of essential oils, infusions, freeze-dried powders or decoctions (extractions), are incorporated into any number of commercial hair care preparations. They are vital ingredients added to shampoo, conditioner, rinse or setting lotion bases to enhance the shade and shine of the natural hair colour.

But these ingredients can be just as easily called for use at home. It is well known that henna has long been used to enrich the colour of red hair; camomile and yarrow have traditionally provided a beneficial rinse for fair and blond colourings; and sage leaves or tree bark were used to deepen brunette tones. But there are also many lesser-known plants that can be used as well.

A word of warning, though. Because vegetable dyes have good staining powers, rather than the penetrating abilities of chemically based permanent and semi-permanent rinses and tints, they can have rather fierce-looking effects on white or bleached hair. If there is more than 10 per cent white in a naturally red hair colouring, for instance, henna can produce a noticeable carrotty look in that sprinkling of white. Better to choose rhubarb, for instance, for a rinse which won't produce such a brightly coloured effect. Also, a build up of henna and other vegetable dyes can prevent a perm from taking properly.

For do-it-yourself at home hair colour enhancers, the leaves, petals or fruit of the chosen plant should be picked, rinsed in cold water to remove dirt, placed in a (non-metallic) bowl and then covered with boiling water. Leave to stand for twenty minutes or so and then strain liquid into a clean bowl ready for use as a final rinse after shampooing. Where the roots and stalks of plants are used, a decoction (extraction), rather than the above infusion, method is better for extracting the required colouring element. Again, rinse the roots or stalks in cold water to remove dirt and earth, cut them up into 1-inch (2.5-centimetre) cubes, place in a saucepan, cover with boiling water and allow to simmer for about fifteen minutes. Allow to cool, strain and use liquid as a rinse.

In *The Ladies Dictionary*, printed in England in 1694, it was written that 'a mixture of bark or oak root, green husks of walnuts, the deepest and oldest red wine and oil of myrtle will turn any colour hair as black as jet'.

From fields, gardens and woods come an amazing range of natural hair dyes. Most of them have been in use for centuries and recipes for their use have been passed down from generation to generation. They are used mostly as rinses that, as well as enhancing the hair's natural colour, give a shine because their slightly acidic properties leave the cuticles of the hair shaft smooth and capable of reflecting light that imparts a subtle sheen.

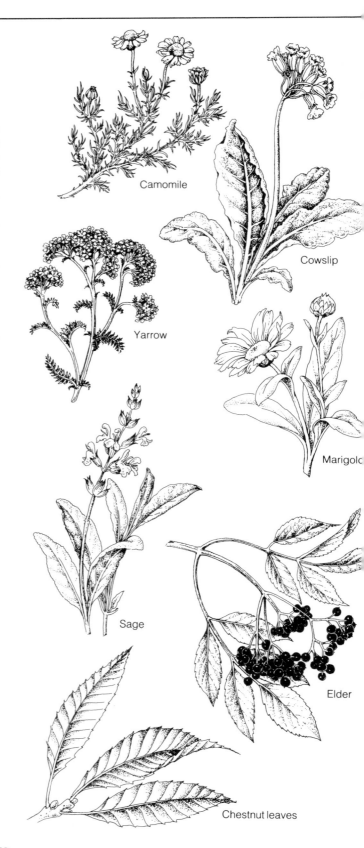

Camomile

Cowslip

Yarrow

Marigold

Sage

Elder

Chestnut leaves

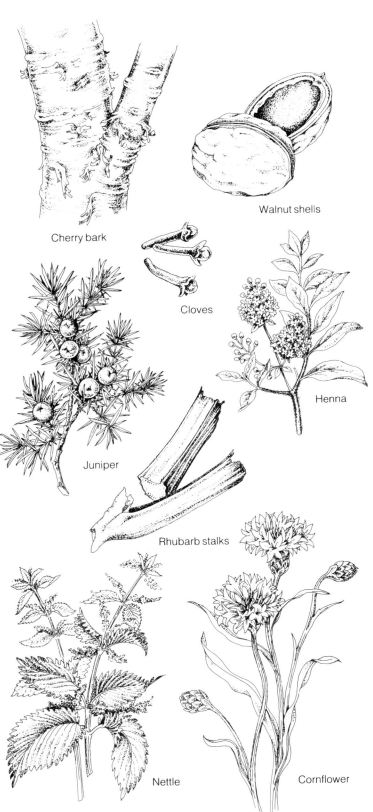

Cherry bark

Walnut shells

Cloves

Henna

Juniper

Rhubarb stalks

Nettle

Cornflower

IF YOUR HAIR IS FAIR OR LIGHT BROWN

Camomile flowers
  A brightening rinse to emphasize the natural
  highlights.
Marigold petals
  Brightens blond tones.
Yarrow petals
  Imparts a golden gleam.
Cowslips (Primrose)
  Lightens naturally fair tones.

IF YOUR HAIR IS MID-TO DARK BROWN

Chestnut leaves
  Deepens the colours and gives a warm glow to hair.
Tea leaves
  Enriches the colour tone.
Sage leaves
  Darkens and helps prevent fading.
Elderberries
  Restores fading colour.

IF YOUR HAIR IS BRUNETTE TO BLACK

Walnut shells
  Gives greater warmth and depth of shade.
Elder leaves
  Enriches natural colour.
Cloves
  Deepens and adds lustre.
Cherry bark
  Gives rich, dark tones.

IF YOUR HAIR IS AUBURN TO RED

Henna (powdered leaves)
  Creates lights, and brightens up the dark red tones.
  The change depends very much on the natural hair
  colour and the time the henna is left on the hair.
Rhubarb stalks
  Gives a richer sheen to natural red highlights.
Juniper berries
  Deepens the auburn tones.
Witch hazel bark
  Adds darker red tones.

IF YOUR HAIR IS GREY OR WHITE

Cornflowers (the petals)
  Adds gentle silver highlights to the white hairs.
Nettle leaves
  Helps maintain even tones and prevents yellowing.

Choosing a colour to suit you

You can change your hair colour almost as often as you can change your lipstick. There are very many types of colourant to give temporary shade changes and enormous variations in shade and tone in the more permanent colourants. But remember the basic principle in hair colouring is that the end result depends not only on the shade you choose, but also on your own natural hair colour. If two women apply the same shade of tint and the natural hair colour of one is slightly darker than the other, the end result will be slightly different. It is the combination of natural colour and colourant that has to be taken into consideration when choosing the shade you would finally like to be.

If you are a woman, unless you are prepared to make radical changes in your make-up, it is as well to choose a shade that has an affinity with your skin tone. It is more flattering, especially for the more mature woman.

The same goes for men, too. Restoring hair that has gone white back to its original dark colour can create a very artificial look, because along with fading hair colour go fading skin tones, and while a woman can compensate for this with make-up, there are not many men prepared to go beyond getting a suntan to add colour to their faces. Better for a man to choose several shades lighter than the original colour and keep to the light to mid-brown tones of a colourant.

A change of clothes and make-up

For the woman who chooses a positive change of hair colour, a change of make-up and probably a change of wardrobe will be necessary. Hair colour cannot be looked at in isolation. It has to be part of a coordinated total look, and a visual imbalance is the result if make-up shades are not changed to complement the new hair colour. Because when you wear the wrong colour – whether in clothes or make-up – which clashes with your hair, it creates a sense of disharmony. Other people, rather than yourself, tend to notice this and may be more aware of the clashing colours than of you as a person.

The colour of your eyes will not alter, but if your hair is a more dramatic shade than it was previously, you will probably need to add more emphasis to your eye make-up to balance your looks. This you may choose to do with very striking eye shadow colours or with bolder definition of the eye shape through liner, kohl or mascara.

Then, to balance your features even further, you might have to alter the shade of lipstick you normally use to tone in with the hair colour or give the mouth an equal emphasis with the eyes.

When it comes to clothes, you are likely to be firmly established regarding the colours you like to wear and will probably find it harder to make a switch in your clothes than with your make-up. It is also considerably more

CHANGING COLOUR CHART

This chart is a guide for you to use once you have decided to change the colour of your hair. Choose the colour – from those presented on the right-hand page – that corresponds most closely to your own natural hair colour. Then, consider the colour you would most like to become – from the choices presented below. Follow the boxes down and along respectively and where they meet you will find advice to help you achieve your desired hair colour.

COLOUR YOU WANT TO GO

Blond

Light brown

Red

Dark brown

Black

YOUR NATURAL HAIR COLOUR

Fair to mousey	Brown and red-brown	Dark brown to black	Grey to white
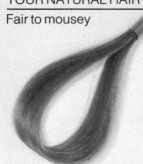	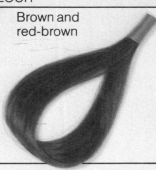	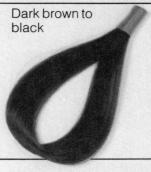	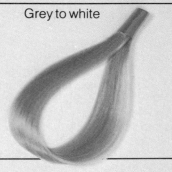
Shampoo-in permanent colourant will lighten up to four or five shades, providing colour tones ranging from ash to beige-blond.	Lighten with bleach and use an ash rinse to neutralize brassy or red tones. The strength of bleach will determine blondness.	Difficult change to make. Drastic bleaching followed by an ash rinse to kill the red tones likely to be left.	If hair is an even, all-over white, just use a blond rinse. If hair is 'pepper and salt', pre-bleach to even out colouring - then rinse.
Semi-permanent or temporary rinse enriches natural colour. Permanent tint in a light brown shade gives a more positive effect.	Enhance natural colour with gentle lightener included in most pale permanent tints or bleach, and use semi-permanent for required shade.	Bleach first and then apply an ash-toned rinse or semi-permanent tint to disguise the brassy tones that can result.	Choose a permanent tint that is designed specifically to colour in grey hair in a light colour tone.
Choose from light, fiery reds to rich, deep auburn in permanent or semi-permanent tints and rinses.	A light copper semi-permanent will enhance natural red highlights, or use an auburn permanent tint to give deeper red tones.	Pre-lighten with bleaching and use a rinse or tint with red tones to achieve shades ranging from copper to auburn.	Take care if the grey is concentrated in one area, a red tint could be too fierce. Choose an auburn shade rather than light red.
Permanent tint or semi-permanent, in tones ranging from a mid-brown to deep brunette, will give as much colour change as required.	Semi-permanent or permanent tint in the chestnut to brunette shade range will give rich, warm tones and colour depth.	Intensify naturally dark colour tones with deeper shades of permanent or semi-permanent tint, temporary rinses or coloured setting lotion.	Beware of going too dark; it is unflattering to skin tones that will have faded too. Choose a light rather than dark brown colour.
A drastic change will best be achieved with a permanent colour that has sufficient depth to give raven and blue-black shades.	The deepest shades of semi-permanent or deep brown to black shades of permanent tint will add the colour required.	Deepen natural hair colouring with a darker rinse or tint to provide the depth of shade required.	Avoid a really deep shade which can give a harsh contrast to skin colouring. Choose a dark brown that will cover the grey.

expensive to change the contents of your wardrobe than it is to change the contents of your make-up drawer.

You will be able to exist with most of your clothes quite happily, especially with the addition of the odd accessory, such as a scarf, large brooch or flower, necklace or belt, in a colour to match or boldly contrast with the new hair colour. For instance, if you've always favoured oatmeal and biscuit tones that have gone well with your mid-brown hair, but now you have taken the plunge and changed to an ash blond, your clothes could tend to merge with your blond hair to the point of dullness. But with a splash of bright red colour, say, the clothes will re-assert their line and style to give a more coordinated fashion look.

Similarly with dark colours. If you have deepened your hair shade to a raven tone, don't wear unrelieved black or chocolate browns. Or with the grey shades: pastel blues, pale greens and pinks are softer and more flattering than bright versions of the same colour.

Matching make-up, clothes and hair is very much a matter of common sense. If you have a flair for fashion it is something that will be second nature to you and you will adapt certain aspects of your looks without even giving a second thought to what you are doing. Usually the fact that you took the decision to change your hair colour is enough to make you re-assess your overall image and be more aware of what does or does not suit you.

Make-up is perhaps the most important aspect when considering colour tones that blend with hair shades, simply because the hairline overlaps the forehead, temples and sides of the face. Also, if you have changed your hair shade because the colour has faded – that is, you have gone grey – then you should realize that your skin colour will have faded, too, and the foundation shade you have always used will need to be adjusted to suit either your paler skin tone or to tone in with a newly enriched or changed hair colour.

CHART FOR CHOOSING THE MAKE-UP TO SUIT YOUR NEW HAIR COLOUR

HAIR COLOUR	FOUNDATION	BLUSHER/ROUGE	EYE SHADOW	LIPSTICK
Blond to fair with ashen tones	Pale beige	Soft pink	Pastel blue/pink/ mauve/silver grey	Cool clear pink with blue or mauve tones
Warm blond with light to mid-brown shading	Warm beige/ pale tan	Coral/light tan	Warm gold/coral/ earth brown/cream	Coral/orangey pink
Mid-red to auburn tones	Ivory to constrast/ beige tan to tone in	Russett/copper-coloured tones	Autumn browns/ olive/khaki/gold	Warm brown/ deep reds/ copper-coloured tones
Dark blond to mid-brown	Pinky beige/ medium tan	Deep coral/ rose pink	Muted browns/ beige/grey/pink	Rosy pink/warm browns
Mid-brown to brunette and black	Pale tones for light eyes/olive tones for dark	Rich pink to deep coral	Rich brown and gold/mid-green/ silver grey	Warm apricot/ coral red
Silver-grey and white	Pink/ivory/pale beige	Soft pink/biscuit	Pastel blue/pink/ mauve/silver/ dove grey	Cool, pale pink/ orchid

Highlighting

If you long to be blond but dread the hassle of all that regular root retouching, then highlighting is for you. Fine streaks bleached through the hair give an effective and natural-looking colouring that needs the minimum amount of upkeep.

Basically, there are two methods of highlighting: the cap method and the foil method. But many different effects can be achieved according to how and where the bleach is applied, whether the streaks are fine or chunky and whether they run through the length of the hair or are concentrated on specific areas, such as the ends, the temples or hairline.

With both the aluminium foil and plastic cap methods, you can highlight your hair from root to tip or you can treat just the ends to give a tipping effect, which is sometimes called frosting or feathering. Or you can just paint on the bleach with a small brush to the very ends of individual hair sections.

The general rule is: the finer the streaks, the more natural the effect because they blend in with the natural hair colour. Also, where very fine streaks are only applied to the top layer of hair, they give mousey, light and mid-brown hair colouring the same kind of lift it gets from exposure to sunlight – the summer blond effect that looks so good with a lightly tanned skin. Because the effect is so natural there is no obvious demarcation line as the bleached hair grows out, just a subtle gleam of light whatever the stage of regrowth, which means more streaks can be easily added at any time.

But, however you put in streaks and highlight, remember it is often not just a matter of bleaching. You may want the hair toned, too, with a temporary rinse or semi-permanent or permanent tint. This can either give a variety of effects by adding bright or subtle colours to the hairstyle, or ensure a natural-looking colour by blending the streaks in with your own hair and calming down any brassy tones that can result from bleaching.

If you are going to highlight your hair yourself, remember you should take a strand test to check that your hair is in good enough condition to take the bleach and to show the degree of blonding you can expect to achieve. Also, use a good conditioner after treatment to counteract any drying effects to the hair.

The foil method

The method of highlighting you choose very much depends on the length of your hair and how precisely you want the streaks placed. If your hair is shoulder length or longer, the aluminium foil method is more effective. This entails covering the strands of hair with bleach and wrapping each one individually in a square of foil. It is a method that allows for maximum accuracy, because each streak can be placed exactly where it is needed. They can be threaded all through the hair, in the under layers as well as through the top layer, which can give more depth of colour especially attractive on the mid- to darker brown shades of hair.

THE FOIL METHOD

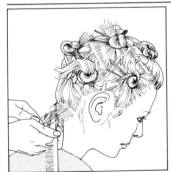

1. Starting at the nape, section the hair into 1 inch (2.5 centimetres) thick partings with tail comb (rat tail). Weave out about 6 meshes of hair.

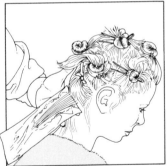

2. Lay the weaved meshes on to tinfoil, apply colour and fold into a small parcel, folding each edge over to the middle, 2 or 3 times. Pinch edge of foil at root to stop colour seeping out.

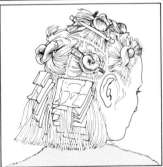

3. Work all round the under section of hair, treating strands at evenly spaced intervals. Repeat process on next section above the first and so on, working towards the centre of the scalp until approximately sixty hair strands have been treated.

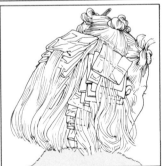

4. As soon as you have finished the application, check development time of first highlight. Processing time depends largely on the base shade of the hair and strength of the bleach, so check at regular intervals. When processing is completed, remove foil from the back first. Rinse off bleach with a mild shampoo. A toning rinse can be applied after shampooing.

On average, fifty to sixty strands of hair need to be treated to give an all-through blonding effect, so it is a fairly lengthy and difficult process to do for yourself. It is far better to leave it to a hairdresser.

The cap method

A quicker and easier method – especially suitable for short hair – that you can do for yourself at home is the plastic cap method. This requires a close-fitting plastic cap, shower cap or plastic bag – or even an old rubber bathing cap – which is punctured with a pin to allow fine strands of hair through. This is coated with a layer of bleach, then covered with another cap or sheet of tin foil while the bleach is allowed to develop. With this method only the top layer of hair is treated and precise placing of streaks is not so easily obtained. The overall effect, though, gives the hair a subtle sheen of blond colour.

Thick streak bleaching

Another effect can be achieved by painting on bleach in wider, bolder stripes. These thick streaks – called flashes, bolts of blond or heavy frosting – can do wonders for lifting a hairstyle by emphasizing the line of a haircut, drawing attention to the fullness of a style at the sides of the face or the top of the forehead or giving an illusion of spikiness to a short cut.

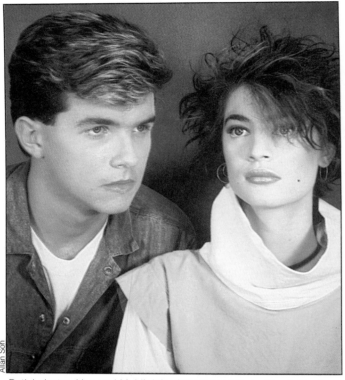

Both hair streaking and highlighting impart natural– looking lightening effects that make the hair look healthy.

THE CAP METHOD

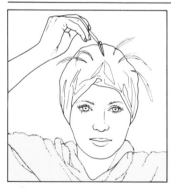

1. Cover head with a showercap or polythene bag, making sure all hair is neatly tucked in. Use a hairpin or crochet hook to make small holes in the cap at 1-inch (2.5-centimetre) intervals, in rows across the head. Pull a few hairs through each hole, keeping the strands as fine as possible.

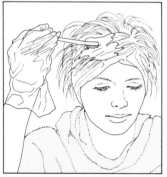

2. Prepare bleaching product according to manufacturers' instructions and apply generously over picked-out strands with an old toothbrush or sponge, making sure all sections of the head are well covered. Then cover with another cap or kitchen foil shaped into a tight cap. Remember that it is not easy to determine exactly where the streaks will be placed, since the hair is obscured by the plastic cap.

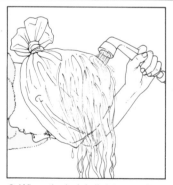

3. When the hair is light enough wash off all the bleach while the cap is still on your head. This ensures that the bleach does not touch any part of the hair not to be lightened. Once you are sure all the bleach is off, remove cap, shampoo hair thoroughly and rinse well.

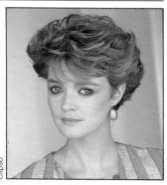

4. You can finish the treatment with a semi-permanent or water rinse to tone down brassiness or add a bright-toned colour. The bleached hair will pick up the added shade, the untreated hair will not be affected. Then set and style your hair in the usual way.

84

Tipping

Tipping the hair with colour is very similar to highlighting, except, as the name suggests, only the very ends of the hair are treated with colour or bleach. Also, the colour or bleach is applied in smears rather than in extremely fine streaks like highlighting.

It is a technique that works best on short to mid-length hair and it is best to have your hair cut to style first and then choose exactly where you want the splashes of colour or lightener to go. Long hair is not suitable for this treatment.

Colour or bleach is used, depending on what shade your hair is already. If it is dark, you will need to use bleach to take out natural colour where required and then follow the treatment with a rinse or tint. If your hair is blond or has been pre-lightened all over with a bleach, you choose the shade of tint or rinse that you want and may be able to get

any effect – from browns and reds that give a tortoiseshell pattern to bright primary colours that give an effective fun look.

Most usually, a combination of bleach and semi-permanent colourant in pink, red, blue, orange or green is used to achieve a fantasy look and one advantage is that, because the hair colouring is meant for fun, it doesn't have to be perfectly applied. You can get away with a look that is, frankly, messy. Another advantage is that, because the bleach or colour has been applied only to the tips of the hair, if you really don't like the end result or are bored with the effect after a few weeks, you can easily have your hair cut to take away the coloured ends.

Tipping is a colouring method that greatly enhances well cut hair. It can emphasize the line of the cut, and can better define the shape and contour of the style.

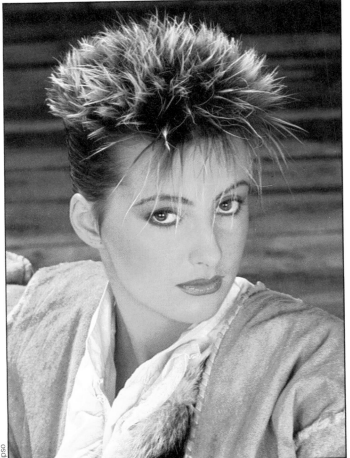

Clipso

Wonderful styling looks can be created with tipping. Strands of strongly bleached hair can give a halo effect that looks particularly good on short hair and, with
brightly coloured rinses, changes of mood and style are quickly achieved. By using several shades of rinse a whole range of colour effects become available.

TIPPING YOUR HAIR

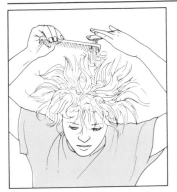

1. Back comb thick strands of hair to the roots all over head and then cover liberally with a spray, concentrating on the combed-out ends.

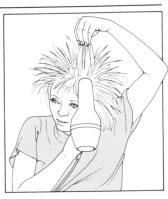

2. Blow dry tips, easing them upwards with the fingers or tail comb, so they stand away in spikes stiffly from the head.

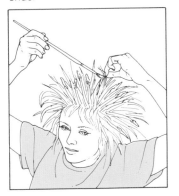

3. Apply bleach or colour mixture to the tips with a small sponge or tinting brush, taking care not to let it drip down the length of the hair shaft.

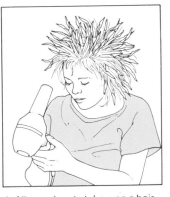

4. Allow colour to take, use a hair dryer with care on low speed, for a quicker development time. Rinse off tint or bleach with mild shampoo and style hair.

Spray-on colour

Hair colour has become as much a fashion accessory as costume jewellery, shoes, bags or make-up. And it is something you can put on and take off with just as much ease with a whole range of 'instant' hair colourants.

These are the spray-on, paint-on, puff-on types of colour, meant to be used for special occasions – usually in the evenings, in party situations – which can be brushed or shampooed out the morning after. They are the temporary colourants, that have been with us for the past thirty years or so, and they are in and out of favour at regular intervals. They get re-introduced in new formats for succeeding generations of teenagers out partying for the first time and wanting to experiment with a 'glamorous' look that can be easily got rid of when it is time to get back into school uniform.

Aerosol spray

The favourite format is the aerosol spray glitter colour, which comes in metallic shades of gold, silver and copper or sparkly bright blue, red, green and yellow – or a multi-coloured mixture of all these shades. The colour comes out in a fine spray of tiny individual flecks, which can be sprayed on in streaks or patches as and where it is required. It may be used to highlight a fringe, add coloured tips to emphasize the shape of a hairstyle or sprayed over the whole head to give an overall glitter effect.

Another trick that can be used with these sprays is to put patterns on the hair – butterfly or star shapes, bows or polka dots. Simply cut out a stencil of the shape required from stiff cardboard, style your hair in the normal way and apply a little ordinary hairspray to hold the hair in place. Allow hairspray to dry and then hold the cardboard stencil flat against the hair just where you want the pattern and, holding the glitter spray about 10 inches (25 centimetres) away from your head, spray liberally over the cut-out shape and surrounding cardboard. Hold the pattern in place with a little more natural hairspray.

The ideal product for use with stencils is a matt finish, non-metallic colour, which gives better definition to the pattern.

Take care when spraying not to get any of the colourant in the eyes. If by accident you do, immediately bathe eyes with plenty of warm water.

Gels

Another form in which these metallic and coloured flecks are found is in gel, intended for use on both the body and the hair. This is especially useful where the colour is wanted to tip a spikey style, because the gel will more effectively hold the hair in stiff shapes than hairspray can. So it is really doing a two-in-one shaping and colouring

job. The gel is simply combed through the chosen section of hair which is eased into shape and left to dry in spikes, wisps or flattened shapes.

Bottle colour

For colour a little more positive you can get metallic or glitter colour in fine powder form suspended in an alcohol-based solution. It comes in a bottle with a brush applicator so it can be painted onto the hair in streaks or squiggles, used to tip the ends or sweep in coloured wings for a dramatic effect at the temples. As the alcohol base evaporates, the powdered colour is left clinging to the hair and can be anchored in place with a fine mist or ordinary hairspray.

Advantages and disadvantages

If the advantage of these colourants is the ease and speed with which they can be put on, the disadvantage is that you have to brush them thoroughly out of the hair before you go to bed at night, or you will have a messy-looking glitter pillow in the morning. Remember that you will also have to wash the comb and brush. Otherwise, the next morning when you do your hair, you will just be transferring the colour back to your hair – and in a random rather than stylish way that can look ill-kempt and tatty. It is probably a good idea to keep a spare brush and comb set for this very purpose if you tend to use a lot of temporary spray-on and paint-on colours.

Also keep a clothes brush handy because one of the annoying things about these types of colourant is that they do tend to transfer themselves to anything you brush against.

Also, you cannot recomb your hair halfway through the evening without ruining the patterned effects. Heated tongs or rollers should not be used while the glitter is in your hair and you have to be particularly careful that all trace of the colour is out of your hair before using any other hair preparations which could cause a reaction.

If the spray gets onto the skin there is a chance that it will cause irritation, since a lot of people are allergic to metal. If this happens, rinse the spray off immediately with some cotton wool and warm, soapy water. Also, as a precaution, shampoo the colour out of your hair as it could quite likely cause irritation to the scalp as well.

Even if you know you are pretty tough skinned and it is unlikely that you would be allergic to the colourant, take care if you have any scratches or abrasions on your scalp that the metallic flecks could get into. It is quite possible that they could cause discomfort at best, and at worst lead to an allergic rash or even set up an infection. You would be advised to resist using these types of hair preparations until the skin is completely healed over.

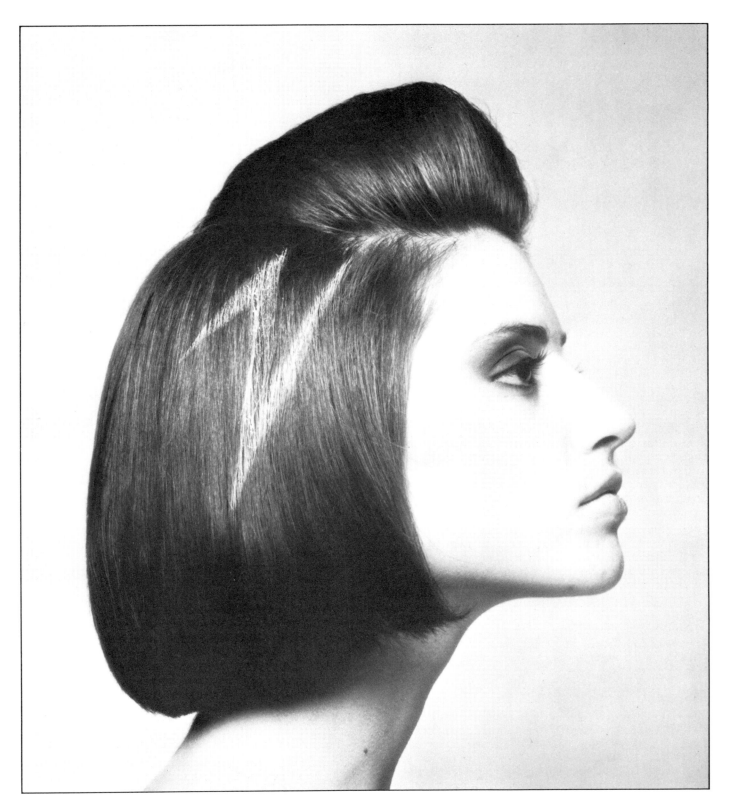

Special effects

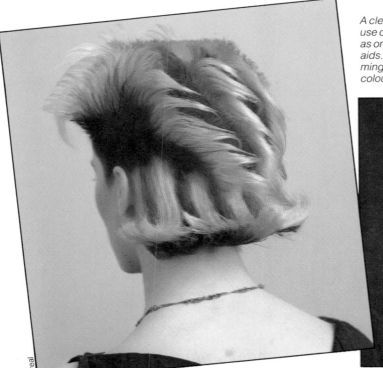

L'Oreal

A clever hairdresser will see the use of special effects in colouring as one of the greatest of styling aids. Blocks of solid colour can be mingled with the hair's natural colour to emphasize a line or curve of the cut, to highlight or contour the shape of a set and to achieve the most outstanding looks for fashion or fun. Colouring can raise hairdressing to the realm of creative art.

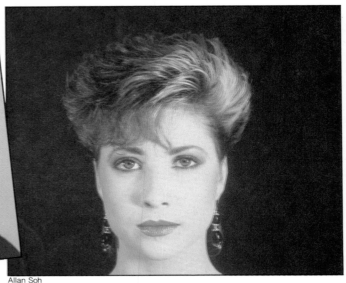

Allan Soh

You have got the world of colour to play with for a change of looks. Whether for fashion, fun or effect, you can call on a wide range of techniques to produce subtle changes of shade or outrageous effects. Whether it is gently flattering or frankly fake, colouring contributes to some of the most exciting looks in fashion.

Generally speaking, most dramatic colouring is achieved on pre-lightened hair because blond shades offer the greatest contrast to bright, zany colours or can be greatly enhanced by the more subtle blond-on-blond tonings that can be so effective.

So if your hair is dark you will need to bleach before you colour. The bleach need only be applied to the sections of hair where you want colour, so it is not going to be such a drastic change as going totally blond and there won't be trouble with root regrowth. But do remember bleach is a permanent process and will show up in your hair until the sections are cut out or permanently coloured in with your own natural hair shade, should you decide a fantasy look is not for you after all.

Professional hair colourists working in hairdressing salons create the most artistic results by mixing tints, rinses and bleaches, using special heat-processing machines and matching the colour to imaginative haircuts. But many of their techniques can be used at home and, because hair colourants are so well formulated and loaded with conditioners, there is not the risk there once was of hair turning into a blond or disastrous khaki —

provided you follow the manufacturers' instructions *to the letter* and don't get tempted to take short cuts.

As fashion trends currently emphasize the colourful in make-up and hair, there are plenty of hair tints and rinses on the market for you to choose from. It was a trend that started in the late 1970s with punk fashions on the streets of London. What was a minority cult among youngsters, competing with each other to produce the most outrageous and shocking look, has been followed by cosmetic houses and trend-setting hairdressers and adapted to suit the needs of a more moderate general public.

Within a very short time the use of hair colour and make-up has become a new art form and brilliant effects are being achieved. It is a fashion look that is mostly confined to the world of pop music, advertising and the media, but toned-down versions of some of the more artistic fantasies are now everyday fashion for the young.

Special colouring effects are fun and an integral part of a fashion scene where anything goes in the pursuit of individuality.

Whether you are after the gently flattering or the frankly fake, find the method you need from among the following colouring techniques.

Halo colour forms a shape of colour that follows the line of your hairstyle. The top section of hair is caught up and pinned out of the way, while the section underneath is laid

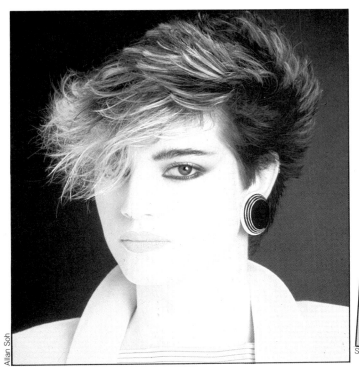

Allan Soh

Selective streaking may look very dramatic and is particularly effective on the wilder, less controlled hairstyle, where it can be used to emphasize the more outrageous aspects of a hair cut or set. It is usually effective on fringes (bangs) and at the temples, because lighter tones of hair emphasize the eyes and cheekbones (like this style on the left).

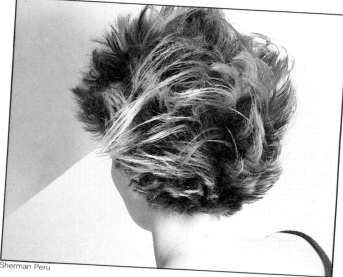

Sherman Peru

over a piece of card shaped to fit around the head. Bleach or tint is applied over the hair on the card, to give a round halo of coloured hair.

Flying colours is a means of introducing a variation in colour to the ends of the hair to blend in with the shape of the style. Different colours are painted on to the ends of sections of the hair, which are wrapped around small sections of cotton wool and left to develop. Five minutes before processing is complete, the colour is combed through the hair length to blend it in gently.

Floodlighting is a technique designed to add a variety of shades to hair which is already coloured. Underneath sections of hair are picked out with a tail comb (rat tail) and colour is applied to each mesh, which is laid over a sheet of clingfilm to avoid getting colour on other sections of hair. Up to five or six different shades can be used to give 'flashes' of colour under the top layer of hair.

Marbling means random sections of the top layer of hair are picked out all over the head and treated with bleach and tint or a bright colourant to give patches of colour in a dappled, marbly effect.

Tortoiseshelling is the opposite of highlighting, a kind of lowlighting which works well on fair to mid-brown hair. Slim strands of hair are picked out and tinted with brown, dark brown and reddish tints, wrapped in silver foil and left to develop.

Speckling can only be effectively done on short, curly hair. Permanent tint is dabbed on to the top layers of hair with a sponge, in quick movements that leave only a little amount of colour at each spot. A temporary colour is then rinsed through the hair afterwards.

Slicing calls for a lightening bleach to be applied to the very edges of the hair, all round the head, to the area around the hairline and at the crown. Then a tint or rinse is put through the hair to give bands of shading.

Special effects like these carry the message that bright all-over colour might not be fashionable. Instead, colourists and their clients like to have a blend of shades which means that two or three colours are run through the hair in streaks, stripes, or shimmers of shade. Where solid colours are used, it is generally to emphasize the shape of a style: colour a fringe (bangs) or put bold flashes of colour around the sides of a head and call attention to some point of the haircut. This technique looks particularly effective where hair is layered very short into the nape of the neck and that section is lightened to contrast with the hair on the crown.

The colours that are chosen tend to ally themselves closely with the seasons.

Plaited (braided) colour is a method of putting zig-zag stripes of colour through the length of the hair, from crown to ends. It looks its best when done on mid-length to long hair which can be twisted into plaits (braids). On short hair it just looks messy.

It is a difficult technique to do yourself at home, so it is advisable to call on the help of a friend to assist you in getting the colour just where it is wanted, especially at the back of the head. You can use a selection of different colours for a variegated effect or you can stick to just one colour as a dramatic contrast to the natural colour of your hair.

By varying the thickness of the plaits (braids), you can create different effects - from fine highlights to solid blocks of colour. But whatever the size of plait, one thing is very important and that is to wind the plait as tight as possible. This ensures that the bleach or colour stays only on the surface of the plait and doesn't spread through the rest of the hair.

If you are using bleach on dark hair, remember that you will need to follow with a colour rinse to tone down any brassiness or provide specific colour tones that you want. The colour rinse should be applied in the normal way after you have unplaited the hair and rinsed away all traces of bleach. Also, where bleach has been used, you will need to give your hair a deep moisturizing treatment the next time you shampoo, to help counteract the drying effect and keep your hair in good condition.

Here, step-by-step, is the way to achieve the plaited (braided) colour look.

PLAITED COLOUR

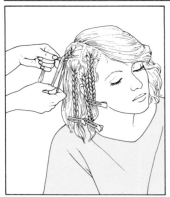

1. Take several slim strands of hair at regular intervals around the head and twist them into several tight plaits (braids) close to the head.

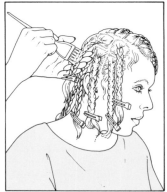

2. Take bright permanent tint for dark hair or a bleach tint for lighter coloured hair and, with a tinting brush, paint the mixture over the top of each plait.

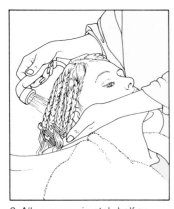

3. Allow approximately half an hour for the bleach or colour to develop, rinse out colour and then undo plaits and shampoo head.

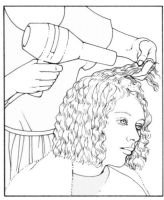

4. Blot hair dry with a towel. Make sure there is no colour left in hair, add mousse or gel if required and leave to dry naturally or blow dry.

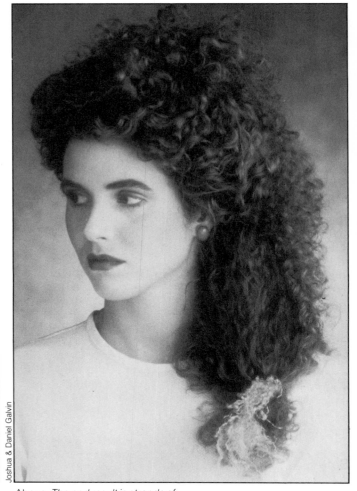

Joshua & Daniel Galvin

Above: *The end result is strands of colour coming through the curls. Lines blur with the natural hair shade to highlight the style.*

Colour problem checklist

Getting rid of unwanted colour can be done, but it is a tricky process and is usually best left to experts in the hairdressing salon who know best how much colour can be safely removed or what new colouring process can be used to disguise the unwanted look.

Whichever method is used, it is generally easier to darken lightened hair than it is to bring a light tint back to a darker shade. When dealing with a relatively simple case of colour removal – if too dark tint has been used and the hair needs to be lightened slightly – a colour reducer will take the hair colour down a shade or two and there is not likely to be a need for re-tinting.

However where the hair has become too dark through repeated tinting and there is a colour build-up, the hair is likely to be left with a certain amount of predominating red pigment from the tint which will be difficult to remove and might need to be disguised by re-tinting with an ash or 'cold' brown hair colourant.

If you want to disguise the fact that you are growing out a permanent colourant, highlights or lowlights will be helpful. On dark hair that has been bleached blond, it is usually effective to bleach a few highlights in to the root regrowth and tone them and the already bleached portion of the hair with a semi-permanent colourant to give an all-over slightly darker shade to the hair. If you are growing out a darker colourant it is possible to reverse the process and colour in brown streaks for a tortoiseshell effect.

Colour reducers

There are products available that will remove the hair colourant that has been used without having any effect on the hair's natural colour pigment. These are called colour reducers and they are applied in much the same way as the original colourant, left on the hair for approximately 15 to 20 minutes to 'develop' and then shampooed out to leave the hair as close to its natural colour as possible.

Bleach-based products

Another way to remove colour is with a bleach-based product which will remove both the artificial colour and the hair's natural pigment. This is called oxidation and is a much more complex process because, unless carefully controlled, it can strip out too much colour and leave the hair with a brassy over-bleached look.

Safety

Before embarking on any form of treatment, it is advisable that both a strand and patch test should be taken to check the product is safe to use and to assess the result likely to be achieved.

Once you have got your hair coloured to the shade you want, you must try to live with it for a while. Although hair colourants manufactured today are specially formulated to be as gentle to the hair as possible, nevertheless, tints and bleaches create a chemical process within the hair shaft that can leave it sensitive or in a rather poor condition. Both your hair and scalp can suffer.

As the hair grows out from the follicle – or root – it is virgin hair that appears above the scalp and any damage that might have been done from too much tinting or over-processing with bleach will be confined to just the portion of the hair that has been treated. The new hair will be in good condition – provided your general health is good and you are not having problems with your diet or taking medicines that can affect the hair.

As the old, treated hair gradually grows out, regular trimming and plenty of conditioning will keep it looking good. But, even so, it is worth giving your hair a rest from colouring from time to time, to concentrate on maintaining its health and condition.

On the subject of safety, there has been some speculation on the dangers of hair dyes causing cancer. Suspicions were first raised in the mid 1970s when an American scientist discovered that ingredients found in some dyes damaged the genetic material of a certain strain of bacteria. His theory, which was disputed at the time, was that if this type of damage occurs the product which causes the damage should be treated as a potential cancer hazard.

Critics of the scientific tests that were carried out at the time argued that feeding rats large doses of hair dyes – equivalent to a human being drinking twenty-five bottles a day – is hardly the same as an application of dye on top of a human being's head every two months. Other tests, also in America, which involved applying hair dyes to the skins of rats, were reported to have shown no evidence of cancer being caused; and these experiments were done at a rate equivalent to a human colouring his or her hair six times a day for an indefinite period.

The problems of testing dyes on human heads of hair is very difficult. Currently, some 100 million people in the Western world regularly use hair dyes and no two people have exactly the same genetic make up, lifestyle or even ways of dealing with their hair or hair preparations. All these factors make it virtually impossible for tests to be undertaken.

However, manufacturers, scientists and cancer research associations are aware that some of the compounds in hair dyes are carcinogenic in animals when applied in huge quantities. The manufacturers are continually changing and refining their formulations to eliminate carcinogenic risks, however slight, and scientists and researchers continue to monitor new products and work to make their use safe for humans.

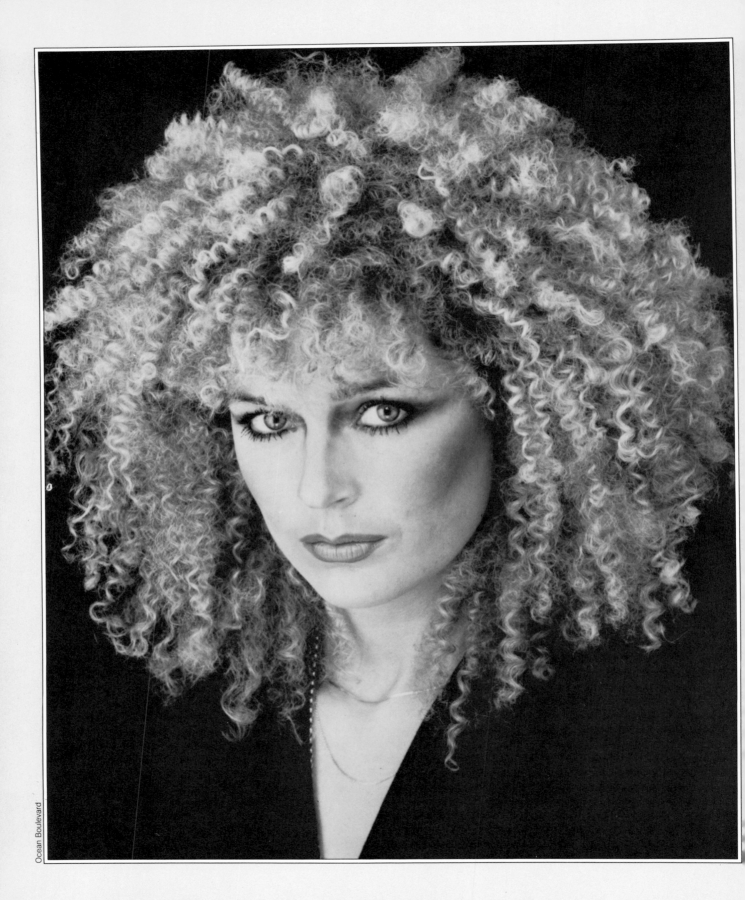

7
Waving and straightening

Whether perming or straightening, there are a few basic rules to be observed. As well as making sure the hair is in good enough condition to take the processing, it is worth having a good haircut first. Uneven, brittle or dry ends soak up straightening or perming solution and can cause frizzy-looking tips and splitting.

If your hair is going to be tinted or bleached, leave two weeks between the two processes. Perm or straighten first, then tint or bleach. Otherwise the perm lotion can strip colour from the hair, leaving a patchy effect. Do not perm or straighten too frequently. It is advisable to leave at least three months between re-processing, giving you time to get the hair into good condition with special treatments and conditioning packs.

For perming to turn out well, both your hair and the rest of you need to be in good condition before you start. If you are unhealthy, for instance, this could affect the results of the perm. And certain medicines and drugs – strong antibiotics or sedatives – make the hair resistant to perm lotions. Also, never perm or straighten if you have any cuts, or scratches on the scalp. The lotion can penetrate the broken skin, causing irritation or infection which might be difficult to heal.

If you are satisfied that none of the above points relate to you then — and only then — go ahead with the waving or straightening process. However, take care!

Conditioning

In between times, be sure to give your hair plenty of conditioning treatments because permanent waving involves a drastic restructuring of the hair and needs fairly strong chemicals to break down the interlinking bonds in each hair and then reform them into a new shape. So it is therefore unavoidable that the hair will sustain a certain amount of damage.

Permanent wave solutions are usually highly alkaline and so rob the hair of its protective acid mantle. This leaves each hair with a slightly swollen effect and causes the protective layer of cuticles to be raised slightly and become vulnerable to tearing or breakage. So it is essential that you use conditioners regularly after you have had your hair permed.

Every time you shampoo, finish off with a conditioning rinse. About every three or four weeks treat yourself to a special deep-conditioning and moisturizing hair pack, either at a salon or as a pre-shampooing treatment at home. You can buy special protein hair packs or mix up your own deep-conditioning oil treatment that will keep hair looking and feeling healthy.

Avoid rough treatment such as backcombing or exposure to harsh weather conditions; do not use a hair dryer on the maximum temperature and avoid heated rollers and electric tongs for the first week or so. They are all hard enough on a healthy head of hair, let alone on chemically treated hair. With a few sensible precautions you can extend the life of your perm or keep straightened hair looking its best.

If a perm or straightening has taken well, it is usually the fault of the aftercare if it looks straggly or frizzy after only a couple of weeks. But if your hair should turn out a mess or – more likely – not the way you had envisaged the new look, there are a few rescue measures you can take.

It is a good idea to have the ends trimmed a week or so after perming or straightening your hair at home because they will probably be dryer than the rest of the hair and could start to split, causing a fuzzy look. If your permanent wave has not left the hair as curly as you would like, rely on regular setting on tiny rollers re-inforced by setting lotion or hair spray to add more curl. Do not be tempted to re-perm or you will just end up with unruly frizz.

On the other hand, if your permanent wave has turned out too curly, *never* be tempted to use a relaxer to remedy the situation. That way leads to damaged and impoverished hair. Instead, remember that the degree of curl will gradually relax a little on its own after two or three weeks, and you can encourage this natural process by setting your hair on large rollers and using setting lotion or spray to stop the hair bouncing back into tight curl.

If you really do not like the new look and quite like wearing your hair short, your best recourse is to go to the hairdressing salon for a cut and a new style.

Permanent Waving

The principles of permanent waving were known to the ancient Egyptians, who wound hair tightly on canes, encased them in wet clay and baked their heads for hours in the hot sun. It was not permanent waving as we understand it today, because, although the hair was set in fairly durable curls and waves, the process was immediately reversible when the hair was wetted. True permanent waving requires that the chemical structure of the hair should be altered from straight to wavy through a process that breaks down part of the hair fibres and then resets them into a curled shape which remains until the hair grows out.

Recent history of perming

Modern forms of permanent waving are a comparatively recent discovery. The first systems, developed in the early years of this century, used heat and steam to process the hair and meant the head was wired up to a fearsome-looking contraption that hung suspended from the ceiling.

Needless to say, the first permanent waves were only available in the hairdressing salon and were difficult and lengthy processes. It was not until the 1930s that scientists made a major breakthrough and achieved 'cold wave' that used special chemicals to break down the structure of the hair without the need for heat. But it was still a complicated process, fraught with difficulty, and considered safe only in the hands of the professionals.

In the late 1940s it was an American company that revolutionized home hairdressing with the introduction of a cold-wave process that was safe and easy to use. The process was called Toni and was the first of the popular home perms.

Perming today

Since then, new and improved formulations have given home perm users an ever-widening range of effects for a variety of hairstyling needs. Different types of curlers, perming rods and rollers add even more choice, and you can now get permanent wave kits for use at home to give hair body, bounce, volume, movement and manageability as required.

You can also get kits to achieve the reverse effect – that is, take curl out of the hair. This is called straightening and, instead of winding the hair round curlers and applying a perm solution, the hair is combed straight and a similar but generally stronger lotion is applied. Combing is continued until the hair has been sufficiently straightened, then a neutralizing lotion is applied in much the same way as for perming. This process, also known as

Clifford Stafford

Warning: Perming and relaxing lotions can damage your hair if not used properly. Make sure you always use reputable products and follow the manufacturer's recommendations. If in doubt, take professional advice.

Curl, curve or wave – all are possible with modern-day permanent waving techniques. With a choice of wave lotion strengths and size of rollers and winding techniques, you can achieve the style you want, because perms are not just about creating curl, they are about giving support and shape, too.

hair relaxing, is more drastic than perming because it is less strain on the hair to shrink it into curl and then fix it into shape than it is to stretch out the curl and fix the hair into a stretched state. It requires greater tension than does perming for curl and so there is a far greater risk of the hair breaking or splitting. It is a process not to be undertaken lightly – and certainly not if your hair is in anything less than excellent condition.

How a perm works

When you permanent wave, you are breaking down part of the keratin structure of each hair. This can be done with intense heat or – more usually – with a chemical-reducing agent which is the basis of the cold permanent waving method.

Keratin molecules in the cortex of the hair are long and spiral in shape, lying parallel to each other with cross-linking bonds between them. The perming lotion acts on these bonds to break them down, enabling the hair to take on the shape of the curler or perming rod it is wound round. The lotion is left on the hair for a certain time, then rinsed off to halt the waving action. Then a second lotion, called a neutralizer and containing an oxidizing agent, is applied to the hair to set it into its new curled shape.

Where the curl has been placed in the hair it will remain until that particular hair falls out. But as the hair grows out from the scalp, the new growth will grow straight as it is naturally, so you gradually end up with hair that is straight and flat at the roots and curly or wavy at the ends. You then have the choice of perming the new growth of hair at the scalp to put curl in at the roots or having the curl cut out at the ends and going back to your pre-permed straight-haired look.

How long a perm lasts depends upon the kind of permanent wave lotion used and your own hair type, as well as the hairstyle you want. If you like your hair to have plenty of curl and have used a perm lotion to give a firm, curly look, you will need to re-perm every three months to maintain the curl.

However, if you have a softer, more wavy look, the regrowth will not be so noticeable and you will be able to leave a longer gap between the perming and re-perming. If you have limp, fine hair that needs the help of a perm to give body or put a little curve into the ends, you will again be using a gentle type of lotion but will need frequent re-perming – say every two months or so – to keep up the desired effect. Because the perming lotion required for this type of process is comparatively mild, your hair will not suffer undue damage by repeating the perming at such short intervals.

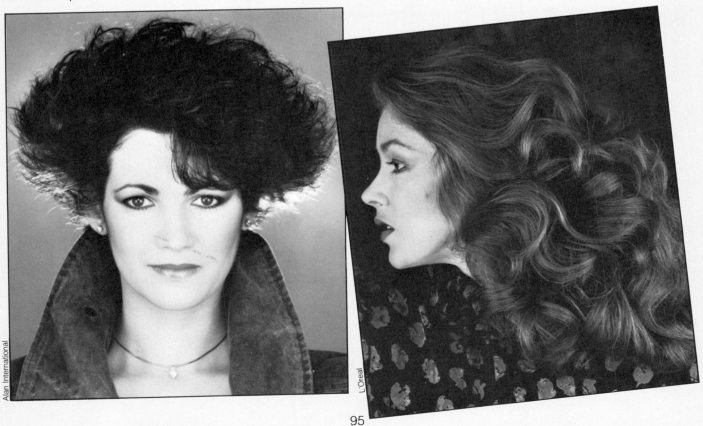

Alan International

L'Oreal

95

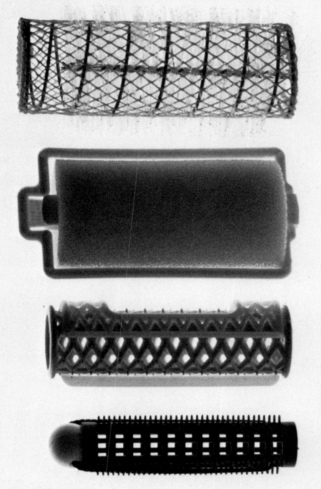

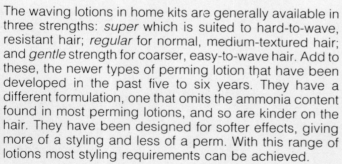

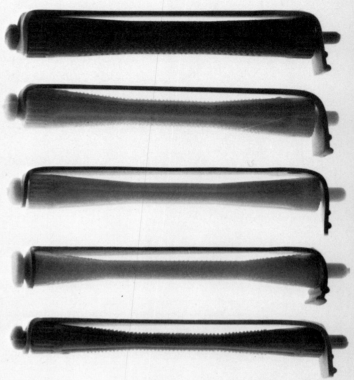

Directly above are thick perm curlers suitable for creating large, curls, and thinner ones which give a tighter perm. Top left is a brush setting roller, which has a metal spring and is therefore unsuitable for use when perming.

Second on the left is a sponge roller ideal for curling your hair while you sleep. Next on the left is a plastic roller with plastic cover to secure. The final roller is bristled with an elastic band to secure.

The waving lotions in home kits are generally available in three strengths: *super* which is suited to hard-to-wave, resistant hair; *regular* for normal, medium-textured hair; and *gentle* strength for coarser, easy-to-wave hair. Add to these, the newer types of perming lotion that have been developed in the past five to six years. They have a different formulation, one that omits the ammonia content found in most perming lotions, and so are kinder on the hair. They have been designed for softer effects, giving more of a styling and less of a perm. With this range of lotions most styling requirements can be achieved.

Perming techniques

Another factor that allows for a variety of hairstyles is the size of the curler or perm rod or roller that is used. This determines the size of curl and the tightness or looseness of the wave and, therefore, is effectively more important than the lotion used. The basic rule is: the smaller the curler, the tighter the curl; the larger the curler, the softer the wave. Perm curlers are usually made of plastic and

they have a waisted shape with tiny teeth along the narrowest part to grip the hair. The larger curling rods tend to be halfway between a setting roller and a perm curler. There are other types of curling rods available, including spiral designs and square shapes for ric-rac effects, but these are generally confined to use by the professionals in the hairdressing salon.

If you want plenty of curl for your style, you should choose a super-strength perm lotion and wind on small perm curlers, unless you have fine hair in which case try regular strength initially. Fine hair will often perm well with regular lotion. However, if the surface cuticles are tightly packed a stronger lotion will be needed.

Coarse hair can sometimes get away with regular strength solution, but experience often shows that a super strength lotion is necessary. You should not use a strong lotion on bleached hair, because it is usually absorbent with porous tips that soak up the lotion. If the tips of the hair seem especially porous, it might help to dampen them with water before perming. This helps dilute the lotion that is applied to the tips, without weakening the

CHOOSING THE RIGHT LOTION FOR YOUR HAIR TYPE

HAIR TYPE	CURLY STYLE	WAVE AND CURVE	BODY AND CONTROL
Fine	Regular strength/small curlers	Gentle strength/small rollers	Gentle strength/medium rollers
Medium	Regular strength/small curlers	Regular strength – but less processing time/ small rollers	Regular strength/medium to large rollers
Coarse	Regular/super strength/ small curlers	Regular strength/small rollers	Regular strength/rollers
Tinted or bleached	Soft perm on premoistened hair or gentle strength/small curlers	Soft perm on premoistened hair/large rods	Soft perm on premoistened hair/rollers
Poor condition	Get hair in better condition before perming	Get hair in better condition before perming	Get hair in better condition before perming

Always play safe when perming at home. If you are in any doubt about the strength of lotion you should use, try the weaker option first.

lotion that is used on the rest of the hair.

A final way of varying perming techniques to suit a particular style is in the way the hair is wound. Most home permanent wave kits give alternative winding patterns in the instructions to help you achieve the look you require. But always take care with the winding. Don't think a tightly wound permanent wave will give you a tighter curl. It will not. All it will do is cause damage to the hair through over-stretching.

Advantages of perming

One of the values of permanent waving is that it can be used to achieve a particular style you want that could not be got with your own natural hair. Selective perming, where just the roots, the crown, or the side of the hair are treated, is best left to the expert. It takes skill to put in the volume, curve or movement just where it is wanted.

In home perming it is possible, however, to tackle just the ends of the hair to enhance a style like the bob where a gentle curve at the very ends is required. You will need to use fairly large rollers to achieve the amount of curving under that is needed, and you will have to take care that the perming and neutralizing lotions are applied only at the ends and not through the rest of the hair. Home perming is at its best for the type of wash-and-wear styles that call for all-over curl that can be simply shaken in to style after shampooing and on short to medium-length hair, which is the easiest to wind. If the hair is too short, it is difficult to catch up the ends on to the roller and you risk ending up with a straggly hairline at the back and nape of the neck. Hair that is too long is also difficult to wind evenly and smoothly and it is often a problem ensuring that the perming lotion and – even more – the neutralizer has penetrated right through the thickly wound meshes of hair to the curler.

Permed hair tends to lose its curl when slept on and when subjected to flattening pressure, but it can be soon revitalized with a light spray of water. An Afro comb, with long widely spaced teeth, is also useful for gently easing out curl and for giving a bit of shape and volume to the style.

97

Straighteners and relaxers

Relaxing or straightening the hair is, like perming or tinting, a permanent chemical process and, as such, has to be tackled with extreme caution. Successfully done, it takes the curl out of hair and is useful for eliminating frizz or giving a sleeker, more controlled, line to the hair.

Chemical straighteners were developed a few years after the introduction of the cold wave process and originally, like early permanent waves, were based on the chemical ingredient *ammonium thioglycollate*. Their chemical formulation was rather crude and they were prone to damage the hair unless used carefully.

Chemical straighteners are applied to the hair which then has to be combed continually or gently pulled into a straight shape while the chemical action has time to develop. This is much the same process as keeping the hair in a curled state throughout the perming process. Unfortunately, because hair breaks more easily when it is wet and stretched, there is a very real danger of damaging the structure of the hair if too much tension is applied during the processing.

Straighteners have improved considerably in formulation since the early days. Because the chemical does not activate as quickly as other types of relaxer, it is easy to check during development time to ensure there is no over-processing. So they are now easier to control and suitable for use at home.

Modern formulations

A newer type of hair relaxer is based on *sodium hydroxide,* which acts faster and is more effective. Also, because it works by causing the hair fibres to swell and break the cross-links that hold them together, it is not necessary to keep the hair under continual tension during the development time. However, because it is a much more powerful chemical, the risk of over-processing is considerably higher and it requires a lot of expertise to recognize exactly when the hair has been processed sufficiently and the neutralizer needs to be applied. This is a process best left to your hairdresser.

Yet another hair relaxer has a similar formulation to the latest 'soft' permanent wave lotions and contains the chemical ingredient *ammonium bisulfite*. It comes in both powder and liquid forms and these have to be mixed together to activate the chemical properties before use. This type of relaxer is kinder to the hair, because it is a less alkaline solution and does not cause so much swelling of the hair fibres. But the disadvantage is that it takes longer to process, so damage can be incurred by the continual combing or pulling of the hair necessary during the processing time.

Most straighteners and relaxers, like permanent waves, come in different strengths; the type used will depend on the texture of the hair and the amount of curl to be removed. Generally speaking, the recommended choice for fine hair is regular strength, initally. As some fine hair is difficult to penetrate super strength may be needed; mild for coarser-textured hair, which tends to be more porous; and regular for in-between hair. Where hair has been previously tinted, choose a mild formulation of relaxer.

Most of these products have been developed especially for the ethnic market to cope with ultra-curly Afro hair, but they can, of course, be used equally successfully on Caucasian hair to straighten out unwanted frizz and curl.

Before chemical relaxers came on to the market, it was customary to use hot combs to smooth out curl. These were heavy iron combs with long teeth that were heated over a naked flame and then pressed through the hair to remove curl. The method is still used today to a certain extent, although the teeth of the combs are now electrically heated. They are quick and easy to use, very beneficial for untangling hair, easing too-tight curls and styling hair for shape and volume. Heated curling tongs can also be used for the same effect but, of course, straightening with electrical appliances like this is not permanent and the curl will return when the hair is damped down.

Whether you have your hair permanently relaxed in the hairdressing salon or do it yourself at home, the straight look will last as long as your hair takes to grow out. That is, after a month there will be about ½ inch (1.2 centimetres) of curly regrowth at the root. But this amount will not be very noticeable, because the weight of the rest of the hair (which will, of course, be straight) will help pull out the curl in the new growth. By the end of the second month, curl will begin to show up. Because it is not advisable to have the straightening process repeated too frequently, it is worth while trying to control the amount of curl at the root area with a hot comb or electric styling tongs (curling irons) for the next month or so.

In home straightening techniques it is best to aim for controlling the curl and turning it into a gentle wavy movement, rather than to try to get the hair dead straight. The waves can be further smoothed out with regular setting on large rollers – but do not set your hair and then go to bed. The tension of winding and the overnight pressure that results from the weight of the head pressing the rollers against a pillow can cause the hairs to split. You can, however, wrap your long hair around your head overnight, which will stop hair from being damaged. Heated tongs can also be used to iron out the curl, but this must *always* be done in combination with plenty of deep conditioning treatment to stop the hair from drying out.

Straightening tends to work best on longer hair styles, simply because the weight of the hair tends to pull against natural curl; on short styles a curly regrowth is going to show up much more quickly.

As the curl becomes more evident you should go to the

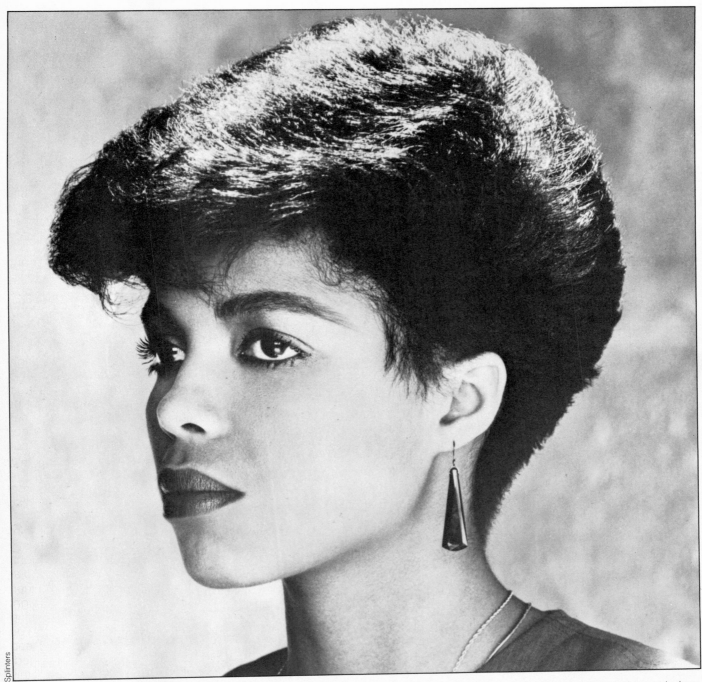

Splinters

salon to have the regrowth treated or, if you plan to do it yourself at home, it is very important to choose a mild relaxer and concentrate on treating and combing only the root area where the hair is curling and not on the already treated hair which should, as far as possible, be left untreated so that there is less likelihood of damage.

Above: *Straightening or relaxing the hair controls the hair's shape and style. A variety of products can create the smoother effects that look so good in ethnic styles. Here, a contoured look provides the perfect balance for prominent features.*

How to perm your hair at home

Once you have chosen the perm most suited to your hair and the type of style you want, and are satisfied that your hair is in good condition and can take a perm, you can proceed with home perming in confidence.

It is a good idea to enlist the help of a friend, because you are likely to find it hard to wind the awkward back sections of hair yourself. Before starting make sure you have all the equipment you need ready for use. Avoid metal which reacts badly to perming lotion, so choose a glass or china bowl for the lotion and use plastic clips and combs. Carefully read through the manufacturer's instruction leaflet so you know just how you are going to proceed and follow it to the letter. It is a good idea to keep the instruction sheet in a clear plastic bag to protect it from getting wet or stained and unreadable.

The initial test

The first stage is to take a test to ensure that your hair and the perm lotion are compatible. This is especially important if your hair is tinted, bleached or has highlights. Take two test curls from different parts of the head, preferably somewhere that is not too noticeable, such as the nape, and, if you have highlights, include a streak or two in your test curl. Section off the strands and wind them smoothly over the curler, just as you would for the perm itself. Pour a little perm lotion into the mixing bowl and, using cotton wool or a sponge, carefully saturate both curls with perm lotion. Leave the lotion on for *half* the recommended time, then partly unwind one of the curlers, pushing the hair towards the scalp to see if the curl is developing and to test the state of your hair. If there is any hint of stickiness or a slimy feel to the hair *do not continue.*

Quickly rinse off the lotion from both curls; apply neutralizer for the recommended time; and rinse again. The hair is not in a good enough condition for perming.

If the hair looks and feels right, rewind the curl and leave to develop for the remainder of the time, then check again. If the partly unwound strand of hair makes an 'S'-shaped wave as it is pushed towards the scalp, the perm has taken correctly. Make a note of the time it has taken to reach this stage, then thoroughly rinse the two curls with warm water. Blot them dry with a towel, and apply neutralizer for the recommended time before removing curlers and rinsing and drying the curls.

If the processed hair looks and feels in good condition and curl, it is safe to commence on the full perming process.

If your skin is at all sensitive it is a wise precaution to smooth a little cold cream around your hairline to prevent the perming lotion from coming into contact with the skin and also to discourage it from running on to the face. It is also sensible to wear thin rubber gloves to protect your hands.

How to perm

Apart from the manufacturer's instruction leaflet, the most important piece of equipment you will need is an alarm clock or kitchen timer, because, with perming, the timing is critical. Never leave perm lotion on any longer than the recommended time; it could severely damage the hair.

Start by dividing hair into sections and, following the basic style pattern in the home perm kit, start winding the hair at the crown section. Keep the winding smooth, holding the hair section taut at right angles to the head.

PERMING YOUR HAIR

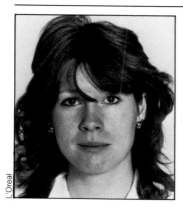
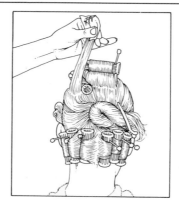
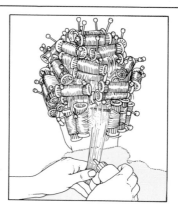

1. Divide hair into sections, starting at the back since it is the strongest hair and it is easiest to deal with.

2. Then move to the top and work down towards first section be careful to get the ends of hair round curlers neatly otherwise they will look buckled at the ends.

3. Put a little lotion on the end of each curler before you wind it on curler. This will ensure that the lotion permeates the hair from the inside of the curl.

The end tissues are important for keeping the ends neatly in place. Fold each tissue around the middle of the hair strand and then slide it to the tip, so the longest ends are enclosed.

Still holding the hair taut, place the curler under the end tissue. Make sure the hair tips do not get doubled back as you wind or you will get a fish-hook effect at the ends. Keep a firm even tension as you wind and finish with the curler resting firmly on the scalp.

Continue winding over the whole head, working down from the crown to the nape, then through the sides and finally to the front section. Rewind the two test curls, even though they will not be processed again. When winding is complete, tuck long strips of cotton wool under the curlers round the hairline, again as a protection for the skin and to prevent drips of perm lotion running down the face.

Pour perm lotion into a bowl and, using a sponge or wad of cotton wool, saturate thoroughly every curler except the two test curls. Leave the perm to develop for the same length of time as in the test, then check on development in the same way. When satisfied with the results, rinse the hair, which is still wound on the curlers, very thoroughly with warm water, making sure it penetrates through the curls. Pat hair dry with a towel and then saturate the curlers with the neutralizing solution, again making sure it thoroughly penetrates through, so that the curl is evenly covered with neutralizer.

Leave on the neutralizer for the recommended time, then unwind the curlers and carefully work the neutralizer through the hair with your fingertips. Rinse thoroughly with plenty of warm water to remove all traces of the neutralizer and blot the hair dry with a towel.

Then set and style your hair in the usual way.

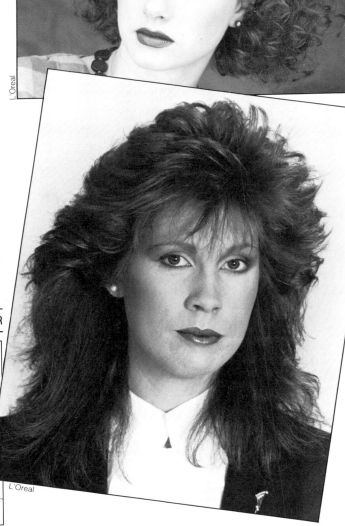

L'Oreal

PERMING YOUR HAIR

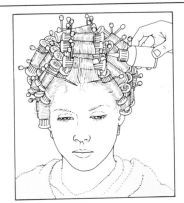

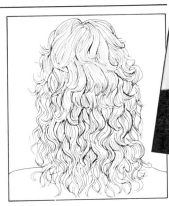

4. When all curlers are wound damp down each curler with permanent wave lotion do not let it run into eyes or on your clothes, if it does wash it out immediately.

5. Finished effect of soft curls on long layered hair. The hair can be washed and left to dry naturally or can be gently blow dryed.

The before and after of perming in photographs that show how body and support can be given to fine hair without making it curl or frizz. Perming is used to heighten

crown hair and control straggling curls. An expert haircut puts the hair into shape and creates a casual but good-looking style.

Perming in the salon

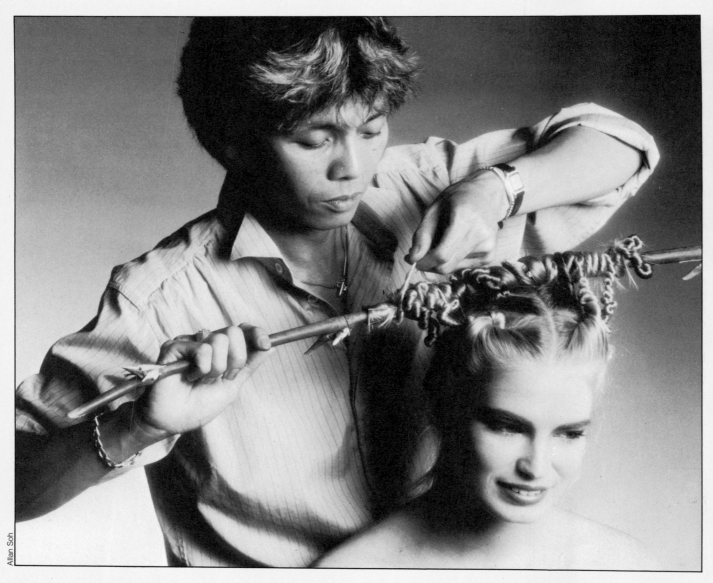

Allan Soh

Today's advanced perming techniques and wide range of products have made permanent waving a very important part of hair fashion. Perming specialists in hairdressing salons can achieve the most amazing results to give body or bounce, tight curl, soft wave, masses of movement all over your head or just in selected areas to complement a particular hairstyle. Perming is a skillful, modern technique that can give the most fantastic looks — both wild and wildly flattering.

Early methods of permanent waving in the hairdressing salon were crude and uncomfortable. A heat process was used and the client was wired up to a machine while the hair was literally 'boiled' into place with a combination of electricity and chemicals. Gradually these elaborate

machines evolved into 'wireless' units whereby metal clips were warmed up on electric machines, detatched and then placed on the already wound and treated curls.

Then came 'tepid waving' techniques which required much less heat and led to the modern day 'cold waving' where the required effects are achieved through chemical rather than heat reaction.

Heat processes are still used in some salons and there are modern-day counterparts of the 'wireless' machine that use hot clamps to help process chemically treated hair on the rollers. There are also 'thermal' permanent wave lotions that create a heat effect by mixing together certain chemicals to build up the temperature of the lotion on the hair and help hasten the development time of the perming process.

But mostly salons rely on the same kinds of permanent wave lotions that are used in home perms kits. Although the professional salon does, of course, have a greater variety of types and strengths of perm lotion to call on.

Modern-day professional perming emerged from the 1970s fashion for the wash-and-wear hairstyle — the casual look that relied on a mop of loosely permed curls that did not need setting after shampooing and could just be left to dry naturally. Since then, salon perming has evolved into all manner of styling techniques, including spiral and stack winding methods, ideal for the very long hair, root perming to give volume and lift on the crown and at the sides, selective perming to put support into a specially shaped hairstyle and many other techniques.

Recently, some men have been wearing their hair longer and have also been requiring a little support for their styles. Afro perms are ideal for many men going a little thin on top because they act rather like a wig and give hair more fullness and body. Root perms put new life into fine, floppy hair, and body waves give control to unruly curls.

Professional advice

When you go to your hairdresser be guided by his or her advice on what is suitable and what is not. But do not let the hairdresser talk you into having the kind of permanent wave that you know will not suit you.

If your hairdresser feels your hair is not in good enough condition to perm, heed the advice. You could suggest the possibility of a root perm to improve a tired-looking hairdo, because there is less chance of the new growth of hair at the roots being in such poor condition as the end sections simply because it has not been around long enough to have time to dry out.

Happily, today's perm lotions are loaded with conditioners to keep the hair looking, as well as feeling, good, and your hair would have to be in really bad condition to prevent you having a perm. Just waiting two or three weeks and having a few hair treatment packs will improve it tremendously.

Always discuss thoroughly with your hairdresser the kind of permanent wave effect you want and make sure that the person who is doing the perm has conferred with the stylist to find out just how the finished style is going to look. Take advice on what kind of treatment you should give your hair between salon visits. And if you also want to have your hair tinted, wait a couple of weeks until *after* you have had the permanent wave.

Living with a new look

Do not be disappointed if you hate the look of your hair immediately you have had it permed. It is bound to look different and will take some getting used to. Also, it might seem a little too curly, but be assured the curls will relax a little and by the time you have had the first shampoo they will not be so tight.

If you feel dissatisfied with your permanent wave, tell the hairdressing salon manager about your complaint. Most salons are proud of their reputations and would rather give you a treatment to help put things right than have you tell friends of their failure.

Although permanent waving frees you from the necessary chore of setting your hair in curls every day, it will need a little maintenance to keep up the style it has been set in. Like any hair, it will benefit from having a regular trim to control the shape.

Perming is ideal for easy-to-manage hair when you go on holiday, but if it is a summer beach holiday make sure you have the perm a good two weeks or so before going away. You will need to let the hair settle down. Also, freshly permed hair is vulnerable to damage from hot sun. When you go swimming — whether in a swimming pool or the sea — make sure you rinse your hair immediately, because permed hair can react badly to both chlorine and salt, leaving it dried out and frizzy.

Finally, if you really cannot get used to the new curls, have your hair cut short to minimize the effect or buy a wig to wear while you are growing out the permanent wave.

Left: *Professionals may use all the modern tools of today's hairdressing trade. Allan Soh uses bamboo sticks.*

Below: *Other hairdressers favour more conventional perm rods to create casual wash-and-wear styles.*

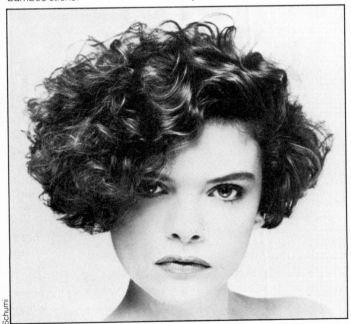

Schumi

Straightening hair at home

The most important factor in home hair straightening is to identify your hair type – whether coarse, fine, thick, or thin etc – and then to match a product to it.

Precautions

There will be reasonably precise indications on the product to tell you whether the product matches up to your own requirements, which can be roughly identified by hair texture and condition. However, before starting on a relaxing process there are a couple of other factors to be taken into consideration: the degree of porosity and the state of your scalp. If the hair shows porosity – which is an indication of poor condition – and if the scalp is suffering from any spots or abrasions, do *not* tackle hair straightening. Wait until you have got the hair and scalp into better condition, until any spots or scratches have healed and the hair is smooth textured. Then you will be able to apply the fairly drastic chemicals needed.

How to do it

Gather together the equipment you need. As with permanent waving, avoid metal bowls, clips or combs. Have a supply of towels, a little cold cream to protect yourself from skin irritation at the hairline, your straightener kit and the instructions – which you should read through carefully and follow precisely.

Do not pre-shampoo or risk irritating and sensitizing the scalp with vigorous brushing or combing before you start. Instead, gently comb through the hair and apply the cream or lotion as instructed, down the hair length from root to tip.

This will require dividing the hair into four sections – with one parting from the centre of the forehead over the crown and down to the nape and the second parting at right angles separating the lower portion of hair from ear to ear. Begin to apply the relaxer cream or lotion to one of the lower back crown sections, working around towards the side and front of the head. Then repeat with the other lower back section working towards the other side. Move to the upper sections, working cream through the top layers from forehead through to ends.

When relaxer has been worked completely through the lengths of hair – upper and under layers – gently pull the hair straight, either using a comb or taking strands of hair between thumb and forefingers and easing them in to a smooth straight line from root to tip

Check for progress of the relaxer: on wavy hair divide out a slim strand and hold at right angles to scalp; when it stretches considerably, hair is ready to be neutralized. For very curly hair, test by holding a small section between finger and thumb close to the roots and pressing it gently towards the scalp. When it no longer wants to

STRAIGHTENING YOUR HAIR

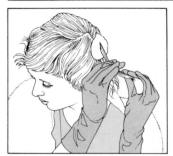

1. Take a strand test before you start. Section off a strand of hair and apply the cream, according to instructions. Leave for required time, rinse, neutralize and rinse again. If hair feels good proceed with treatment.

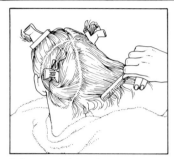

2. Section hair into four quarters, parting from forehead across crown to nape and separating under section across head below base of the crown.

spring away from the scalp, the curl is sufficiently relaxed and is ready for rinsing.

Start rinsing where the first application of lotion was made – at the lower back section of the head. Work quickly, using plenty of warm flowing water to rinse out the relaxer. Work up towards the top of the head, over the scalp towards the hairline, keeping the fresh water streaming through the hair lengths. Blot gently dry and then rinse again, to make sure that all traces of the relaxer have been removed from the hair.

Keep hair in a straight position over the sink and apply the neutralizing lotion. Work gently through the strands – with a comb or between fingers and thumb for the time specified on the instructions in the pack. Then rinse thoroughly until all traces of the neutralizer have been removed. A mild shampoo can be used between the relaxing and neutralizing stages, but this should not really be necessary if plenty of warm water is used to thoroughly rinse out all traces of the product.

Blot hair dry with a towel, being careful not to rub or tangle as you do so, and then set the hair dry on rollers or gently blow dry using the lowest temperature setting on the hairdryer.

Try a deep conditioning pack about once a month and a rich cream conditioner every time you shampoo – paying particular attention to the tips of your hair. Do not repeat the straightening process for another four or five months and then only if you are sure that your hair is well conditioned enough to take it. It will probably be as well to have the ends trimmed to remove any dry porous tips that might drink up the relaxer before repeating the process.

Look after your hair well between straightening sessions. Encourage a smooth line with gentle combing and setting on large rollers.

STRAIGHTENING YOUR HAIR

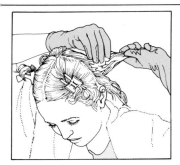 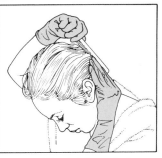 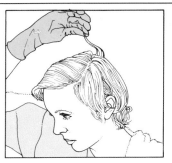 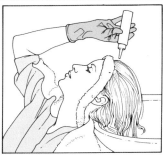

3. Pin upper layers of hair out of way and begin application of cream or lotion on bottom quarter section. Work cream well into the hair length with fingertips and then begin on the next section.

4. When all the hair is treated, gently comb through the hair, pulling it into the straightened shape. Continue combing and gently stretching hair for recommended processing time.

5. Test development by loosening a slim strand of hair, holding it at right angles to scalp and gently pulling. Then push root section towards scalp and, if it does not spring back into curl, the hair has developed sufficiently.

6. Thoroughly rinse hair and then, being sure to keep the hair in its stretched state, apply neutralizer. Comb and pull hair into a straight line for the time recommended. Rinse thoroughly, blot dry and set in usual way.

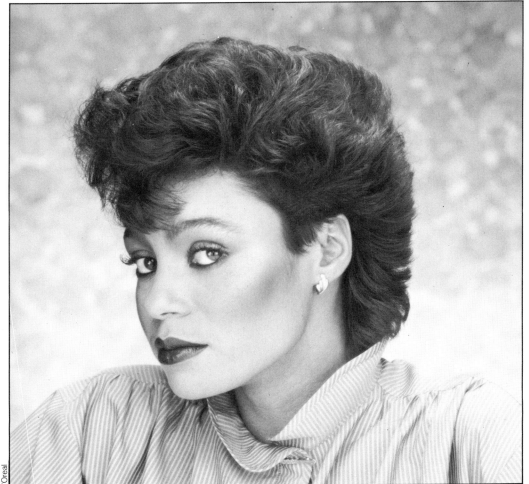

L'Oreal

Straightening is hard to do by yourself; try to get a friend to help. Follow maker's directions, do not cut corners, try to avoid getting lotion on ears or face. Follow the time stated; never leave it on an extra few minutes or your hair might be irretrievably damaged. Condition well after neutualizer. Try not to pull on hair too much while styling it dry.

> **Warning:** Perming and relaxing lotions can damage your hair if not used properly. Make sure you always use reputable products and follow the manufacturer's recommendations. If in doubt, take professional advice.

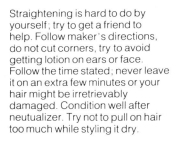

Left: The finished look is smooth, although there is still plenty of movement and body to make the style interesting. Often, hair that has been straightened needs to be set on rollers to provide curve rather than curl and replace the body that has been taken away with the curl.

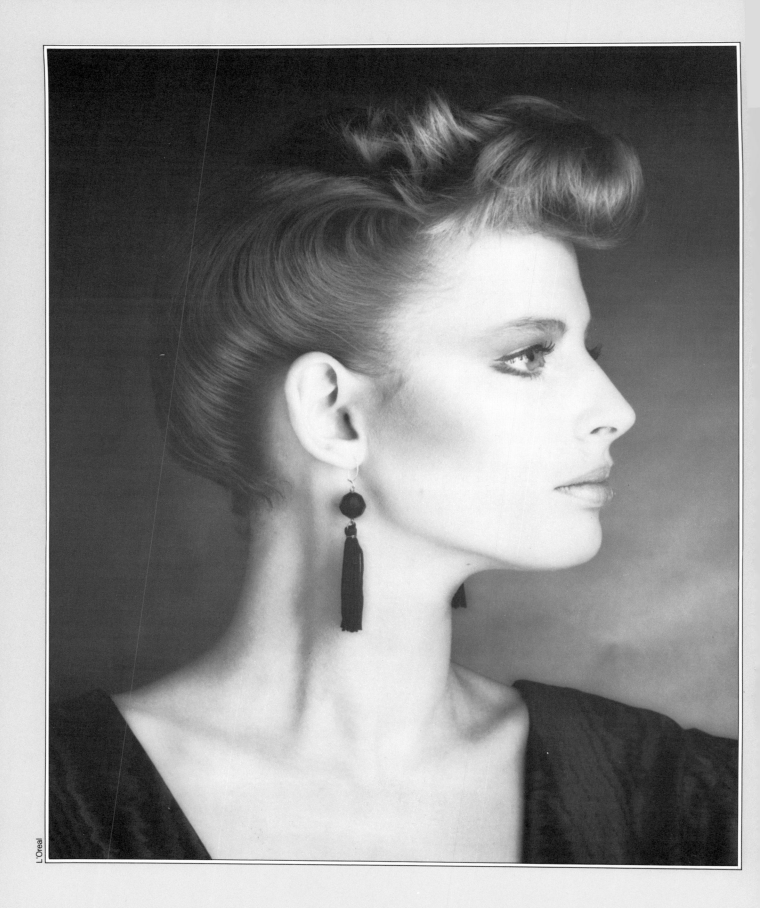

8
Dressing up hair

Hair is the most marvellous natural fibre. It can be treated as though it were a fabric and can be cut, coloured, shaped and moulded into almost any style. Even though it may be dressed in a very simple way, good-looking hair always has style.

Like make-up, your hairstyle should emphasize your good features and minimize your bad ones. It should work for your benefit and be part of an overall look that takes in your clothes and cosmetics, fashion accessories and jewelry. This means you will want a style that is adaptable which can be changed in much the same way as you would want to change your clothes. It will also need to be changed gradually as fashion trends emerge, because it is no good finding the style that suits you perfectly and then sticking to it forever; nothing can date a person quite so much as an old-fashioned hairstyle, so make sure that your style evolves to suit the current mode, as well as your hair's length and texture.

When it comes to fashion, however, in order to look your best you should try to achieve a 'total' look whereby clothes and hairstyle complement each other. It means you will probably need to adapt the way you dress your hair according to the season. The clothes you wear in summer are going to be quite different from your winter wardrobe — and your hairstyle should reflect this.

It is not always easy to know instinctively what style will suit you best and it often helps to enlist the aid of an expert — a hairdresser — who can assess your hair type, study your face shape and come up with a style that matches one to the other. The trouble is that, unless you are a regular client, which means going to the hairdresser at least once every month, your hairdresser is unlikely to know much about your lifestyle — and your lifestyle is a really important factor to take into account when choosing a hairstyle.

A hairstyle can tell other people a lot about you, your personality and your interests. Co-ordinated with the clothes you wear and your make-up, your hairstyle is a major contribution to your total look.

Men should adopt the approach described above when choosing a hairstyle. For them, fashion sometimes changes very quickly — with switches from short to long hair back to short hair again being counted in years rather than tens of years. Very often, once they have found a suitable hairstyle — which may be when they are fairly young — men *never* change their hairstyles. Remember, what is suitable when you are young is very probably not at all suitable when you are older.

Swift changes of hairstyle also apply to children, although fashion does not make such an impact on their styling possibilities, perhaps because fine hair is fine hair in any era and there is only so much that can be done to shape and cut it into style in a child's very early years and even later.

By the time the texture of hair starts to change at the age of five or six, a few styling changes become possible. The choice is still limited because it is unwise to add curl in the form of a permanent wave — no matter how mild the perming lotion, it is still a harsh chemical process which young hair just cannot tolerate — and adding colour is precocious, as is any kind of over-elaborate styling. So children tend to have either the basic 'pudding-basin' (bowl) type cut that adds weight and strength to the ends of fine hair, or, in the case of little girls, long, straight or ringlet-curled styles.

There are many more hairstyles that women can use to alter their looks. These can range from a subtle change that enhances an everyday hairstyle for evening, or a bold and dramatic change that dresses up the hair for a gala occasion.

The use of false hair and fashion accessories, the basic skills of styling and the desire to look right for any occasion can all play a great part in making hairdressing versatile. Above all, your hairstyle should always feel comfortable, and be a style you feel at ease with.

Find out what your ideal style is by experimenting with your hair and observing other people. Try different styles — even if at first you only wear them around the house and don't dare to venture out in public. Look to see how your friends and contemporaries are wearing their hair, then copy or adapt their styles until you're confident you have found the style that best suits you.

The versatility of hair

The length of your hair is going to be a major factor in the style you wear and its possible versatility. You don't always have a choice if you have the type of hair that is thin and does not grow very long because of poor health.

Long hair can look lovely when it is sleek and straight. If this is the effect you're after, but actually have naturally curly hair, you may need to set it on rollers while it is wet and then allow it to dry under a hot dryer, which can take up to a couple of hours depending on its thickness. This is fine, as long as you don't do it too often. Remember that the act of stretching and winding wet hair around a roller can break the hair and fierce heat from the dryer is equally damaging. If your hair is straight and long, but you want it to look curly, a perm is probably less harmful than frequent roller setting. Long hair is only beautiful if it is in perfect condition!

The pictures show you just how different long hair can be made to look and how various styles can be used to adapt to different needs. But whether you wear you hair short, medium or long you can always inject glamour into your hairstyle by dressing it up. Obviously, long hair gives most scope for change. Chignons, French pleats, ponytails and plaits (braids) produce an instantly different look to long hair and are fairly easy to achieve. They are suitable for a range of occasions, from the sporty to the *soignée*, and will see you through a wide range of daytime activities.

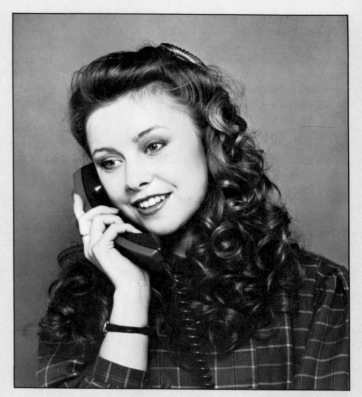

For evening wear, long hair can be dressed up with ribbons, fancy plaits (braids) and elaborate false curls. Jewelry can be added in the form of sparkling clips (barrettes) and colourful side combs. It can stretch the limits of a hairstylist's imagination or be worn in simple but sophisticated lines you can easily achieve yourself.

Medium-length hair is often the most flattering and easiest to keep neat if it is sufficiently long to be caught up into a pleat or chignon. Worn loose it probably needs more care than either long or short hair, with regular cutting to hold its shape and to give it a style that can be adapted to suit the particular mood and occasion.

It is not quite so easy to make dramatic alterations to short hair, but with some imaginative brushing and gelling, some skilful backcombing and the judicious use of hairspray, a switch of parting or change of fringe (bangs), you can soon create a new look. Also, short hair has the advantage of being easy to wash and quick to dry, so you can experiment with glitter sprays, crazy colours and paint-in streaks and shapes, secure in the knowledge that you can easily get rid of them if they don't suit and start all over again with another idea.

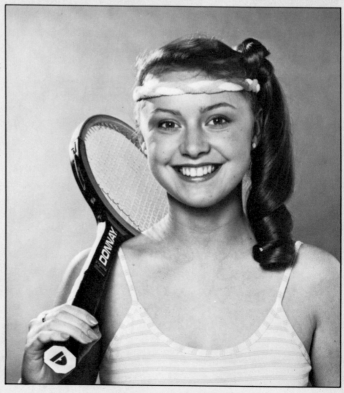

Hairpieces still add tremendously to the versatility of a hairstyle, whether it is short or long. It is best to stick to the length of hair that suits you best for everyday wear and call on the latest fashion accessories to add versatility for a more expansive evening style.

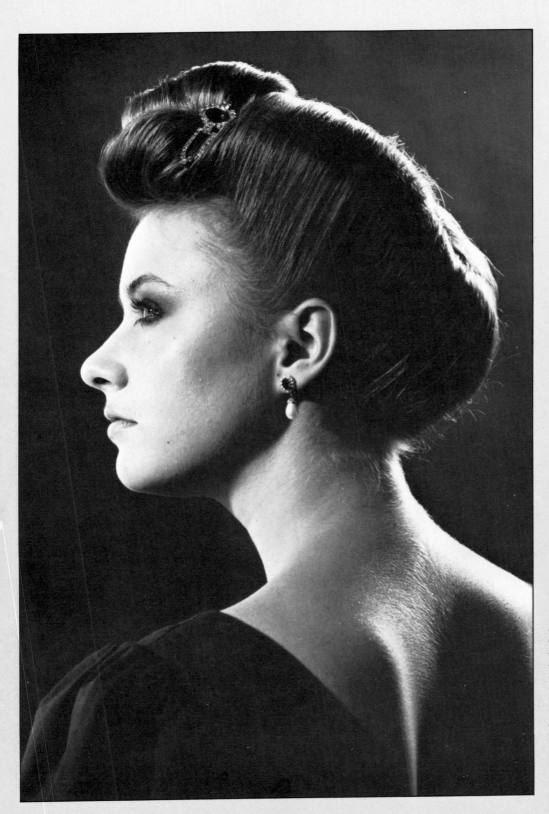

Long hair can be sporty, chic or casual, depending on how it is styled. Dressed up on top of the head it almost invariably creates a look of elegance and glamour; allowed to hang loose, the connotations are vivacious and charming; caught back in to a ponytail or bunch at the side, long hair creates a young and pert look. Judge for yourself with these three styles – each dressed on the same model – just how much hair can change looks and personality.

Deciding on style

It is your hair that sets your style. When your hair is looking its best you feel well dressed and confident, but if it is not up to scratch you can feel drab and dowdy. So it is important to choose the right hairstyle, the one that best suits the type and texture of your hair and the size and shape of your face and figure.

This is where you can benefit from professional help. A hairdresser has the training and experience to know how different types of hair behave, to know where and when a permanent wave can reinforce the hairdo or whether skilled cutting can give the support your style requires. Go to a salon and have your hair done by an expert; ask questions and find out as much as you can about your

hair's possibilities and limitations. Listen to and be guided by the advice you get – after all you will have paid good money for it.

In matters of personal preference, however, you will undoubtedly know best. You know the demands of your lifestyle, the requirements your work imposes and you are the one that has got to live with your hairstyle. So take all this into consideration, too, and, with the help of both objective and subjective viewpoints, make your choice.

Sometimes the limitations of your hair dictate the kind of style you should have. If your hair will not grow long without splitting and is becoming wispy-ended, don't try to grow a long, flowing mane. Instead, stick to a medium-

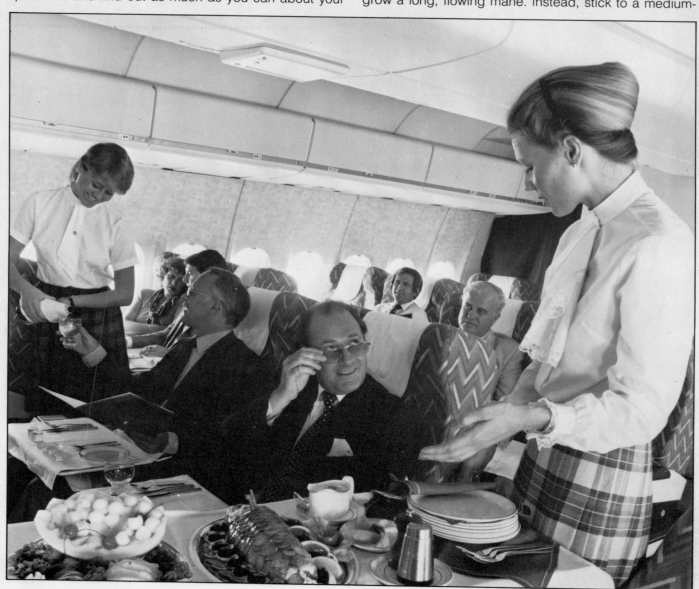

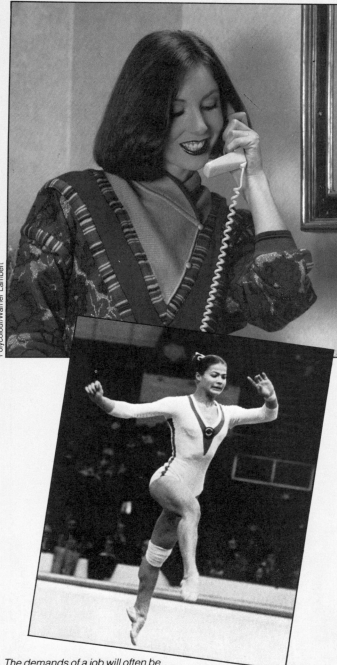

The demands of a job will often be reflected in your hairstyle – whether you are an air hostess, housewife or gymnast, as pictured here. They are demands that frequently call for good grooming and a neat appearance. Make sure your hairstyle matches these criteria with good hair cuts and conditioning treatments. Then consider style and make compromises between what is needed and what personally suits you. It is a good idea to go for simplicity rather than elaborate styling. All these styles demonstrate how neatness and a good workaday look are achieved.

length look that will approximate as closely as possible to the long-haired style you covet.

Like most things connected with looks or fashion, there are a few ground rules to be observed. Be sure that, if you change your hairstyle, it suits on different personal levels, as well as being suitable to your hair type and texture.

For instance, consider your age. Do not go in for pigtails and bunches if you are anywhere near past the first flush of youth; you run the risk of looking ridiculous. Similarly, if you are mature in personality as well as years, a little-girl 'Alice in Wonderland' style would be the wrong choice.

Conversely, avoid sophisticated French pleats and chignons if your clothes and personality are young or on the sporty side – the two images just do not mix. This ground rule is really just a matter of common sense and instinct should tell you what you can and cannot get away with.

Look out for new styling ideas. Be adventurous and experiment with styles to see what adaptations can be made to the basic line; follow fashion and see if any modifications of the current trend can be incorporated in to your style.

Make sure your hair is in good condition by using regular hair care treatments. Have regular trimming and make your hair a trademark of your looks.

A working hairstyle

When it comes to work, being able to adapt your hairstyle to suit different occasions is a great advantage if you have the kind of job that calls for a formal or tailored look from nine to five and if you in your own time like to sport a more casual or fun look. In this case, you would probably do better with medium to long hair that can give you the necessary adaptability.

The style you wear may have to meet certain restrictions imposed by the job you do. It may be a question of hygiene, if you work in the catering trade, or safety, if you work with machines, which means that your hair must be worn short or tucked out of the way. This precaution dates back to World War 2 when the young factory girls who emulated the long hair-over-one-eye bob of film star Veronica Lake were made to wear their hair in nets after a series of tragically disfiguring accidents which were caused by loose hair getting tangled up in moving parts of machinery.

It may be that your job involves wearing a uniform with a cap and certain styles do not look good with it. Or it may be that a short haircut is obligatory.

Usually, there is a way round the difficulties. It is a matter of compromise that can be resolved with an adaptable and versatile style to enable you to lead one life from nine to five and another, completely different, life after working hours.

Putting your hair up

'Putting your hair up.' That is a phrase with connotations of being grown-up, glamorous and sophisticated. In fact, putting your hair up is often a means of keeping your hair tidy and out of the way.

One thing is for sure, and that is that putting up your hair can make a radical difference to your looks. Success often depends on the sheer weight of long hair. If it is thick, and you have got plenty of it, you might have difficulty in keeping it in place on top of your head, whereas long, fine hair will present no such difficulty. However, with the range of hairdressing preparations now available, you can reinforce the old pins, combs and styling techniques with gels, mousses and hairsprays to help you hold the hair safely in place.

For long, thick hair a pretty and simple French pleat style will suit most face shapes and, being anchored at the back rather than the top of the head, will stay in place well. For this type of hair, a chignon, especially when it is pinned at the nape of the neck, can be safely managed and will look very tidy.

For long, fine hair, a 'cottage loaf' style, with the hair wrapped up neatly in a bun on top of the head, can look stunning on the right face, and can look equally good dressed in a casual style or with a formal finish. This style will look after the problem of fly-away hair; keeping it contained and controlled.

Fine hair put up sometimes look very tatty. You can pad it up by adding a made-up roll, consisting, for example, of cotton wool, a pin cushion (without pins!) or almost anything soft and bouncy. Grip in to place at the centre of where the hair will be placed and roll sections of hair over the extra padding until that is no longer visible and all the hair has been fitted into place.

A loose style caught back at the side with combs gives the right kind of fine, curly hair a look of understated elegance.

A French pleat, ideal for medium-length hair, can be positioned either side of the crown. This style is particularly suited to women who very much want a definite style rather than a wild mane.

For coarse, medium-length hair, what could be better than one thick plait (braid) hanging down the nape of the neck? Fine, medium-length hair, however, would be better suited to side bunches or Bo Derek-type braiding; to achieve the latter, however, you will need plenty of time!

Short hair can be moulded into upward lines with gels and brushed back to give lift at the roots and the impression that the hair is dressed 'up'.

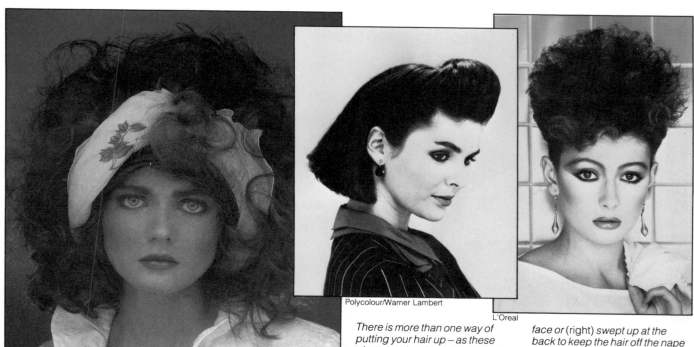

Sherman Peru

Polycolour/Warner Lambert

L'Oreal

There is more than one way of putting your hair up – as these photographs clearly illustrate. It can be caught up with a scarf or turban to enhance a tousled style (see left) or to tidy it up; it can be caught up just at the front (centre) to keep the fringe (bangs) off the *face or (right) swept up at the back to keep the hair off the nape of the neck and balanced with a high-piled crown. It can be drawn back to look supremely sophisticated (opposite) and glamorous enough to grace any gala occasion.*

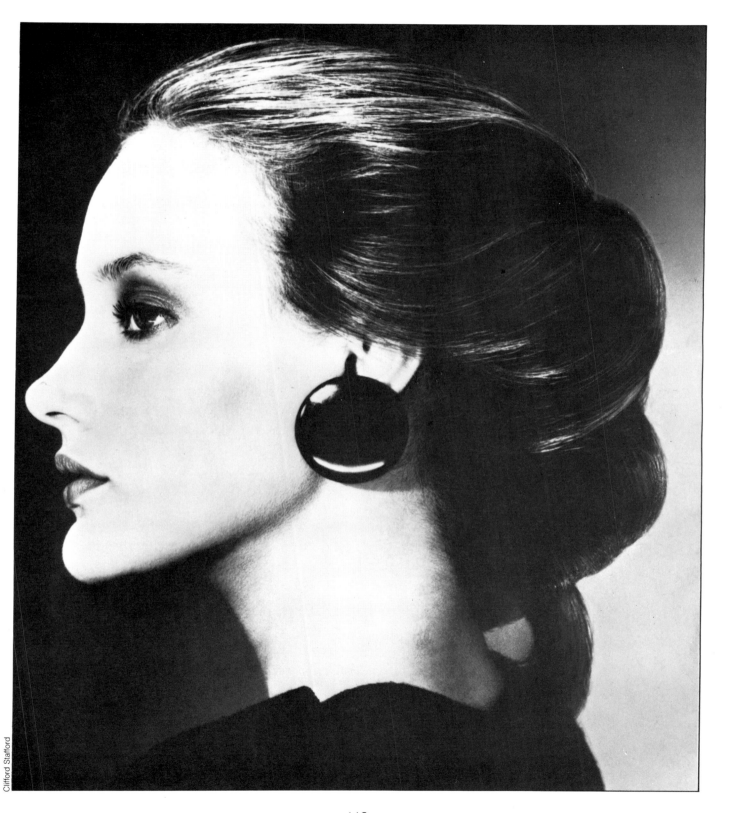

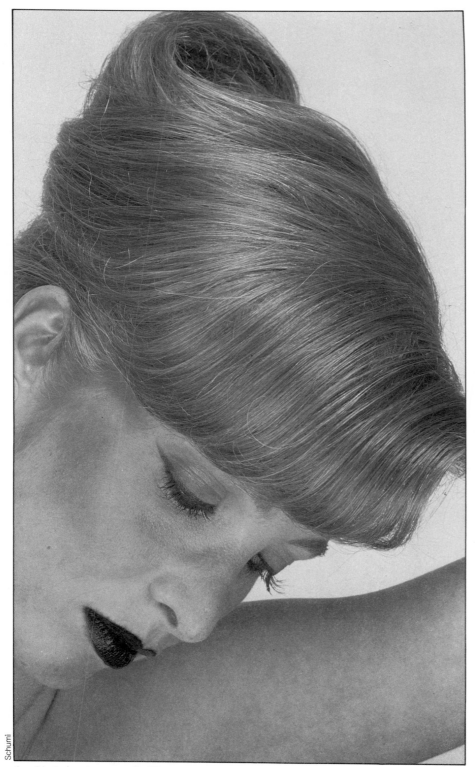

A swirled-round open- ended French pleat for styling elegance which makes the most of long hair.

A FRENCH PLEAT

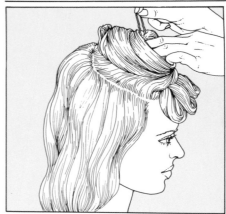

1. First divide the hair into 2 sections. A square is sectioned off at the top of the head. Pin this hair out of the way.

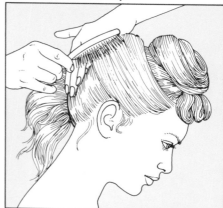

2. The hair at one side of the head, from the temple to the nape, is brushed over to the other side of the head.

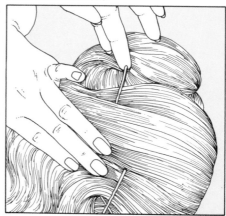

3. This section of hair is then pinned to the head at the top and bottom, down the middle of the back of the head.

A FRENCH PLEAT

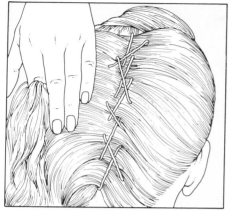

4. A criss-cross pattern is most effective in ensuring that this section is held securely. All of the hair is now gathered together.

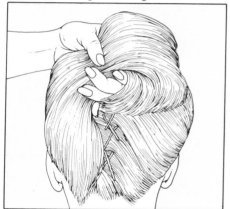

5. The loose hair is brought over to the middle of the head - make sure you don't leave any behind.

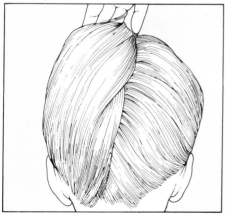

6. Twist the hair up and round to cover the pins that are securing the other side, tuck the hair under and pin it neatly.

A SIMPLE BUN

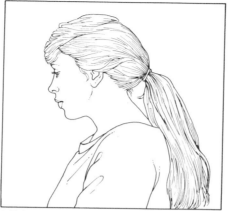

1. Take hair back and catch it in a band, or fix your hair piece securely over the ends of your hair.

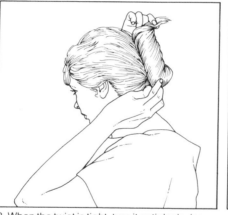

3. When the twist is tight, turn it anticlockwise round the band at base of hair piece until only a little hair is left loose.

Right: *Modern-day versions of that old fashion favourite of the 1940s – the snood. Today, snoods come decorated with beads and glitter, ready for glamorous evenings, and are not only worn to catch up all the hair at the back of the head. They look elegant and effective, worn at the front or at the side of the head to cover neat chignons, and have become fashion accessories in their own right.*

A SIMPLE BUN

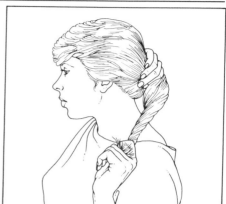

2. Twist the length of hair clockwise as you would a skein of wool keeping hold of the end to stop it unravelling.

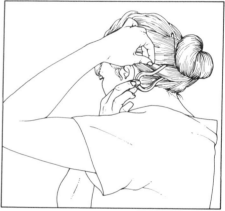

4. When the hair is wound round, secure the end with grips or put several long pins in to stop it unravelling.

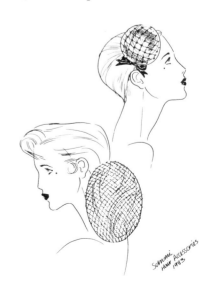

Schumi Hair Accessories 1983

Schumi

115

A ROLLED CHIGNON

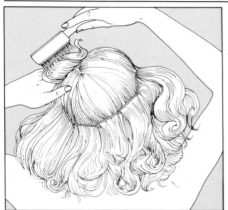

1. Make a small parting above left temple. Comb in the top section of hair. Place grips around crown to form a skull-cap.

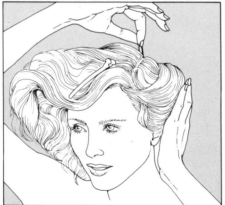

2. Start from left. Roll up a section of hair. Pin this just above the circle of grips at the lower crown.

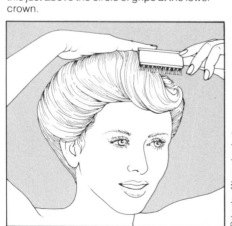

3. Continue this around the whole head. Gently comb through the roll in order to get rid of the sectioned look.

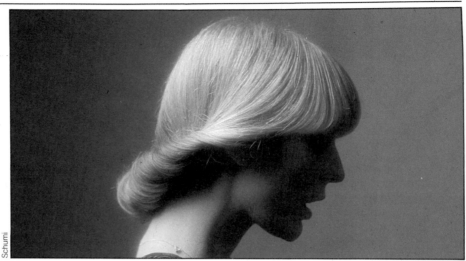

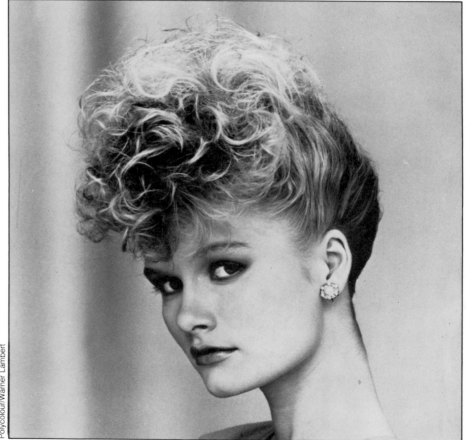

Schumi

Polycolour/Warner Lambert

Simple, understated elegance (above) *or teased-up curls* (below), *show how widely contrasting styles can be suited to the individual.*

A WOVEN CHIGNON

A WOVEN CHIGNON

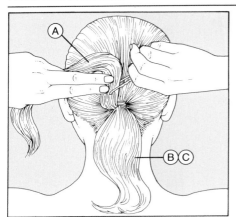

1. Brush your hair into a ponytail at the nape, section it into three and leave two hanging loose. Pin the left hand section **A**, as shown.

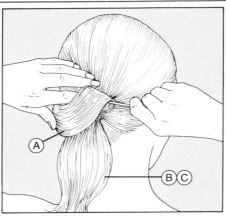

2. Twist **A** back towards the nape, tucking the ends under so that they point down. Pin **A** above the elastic band.

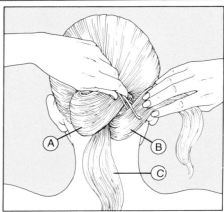

3. Divide the hair that is loose into two equal parts. Take the right hand section **B** up to the right towards the ear and pin it.

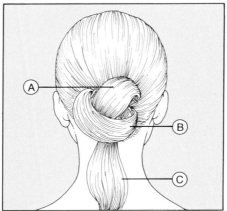

4. Take **B** back, over to the left, so that it crosses over the top of **A**. Pin **B** under its loop, so that the pin is hidden.

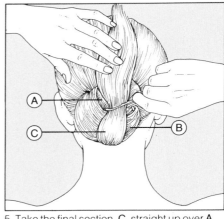

5. Take the final section, **C**, straight up over **A** and **B** and pin it under the first loop, **A**.

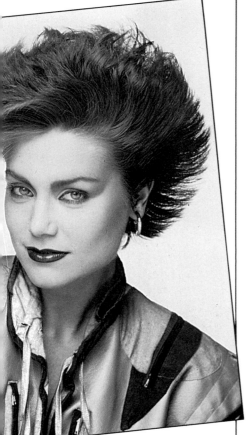

Above: *A simple off-the-face style, feathered at the ends and set with gel or hairspray is adaptable for any occasion.*

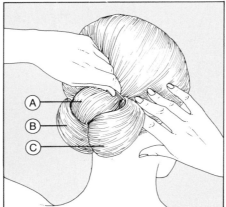

6. Then take **C** over to the right of the head and tuck the ends under, as for **A** and **B**.

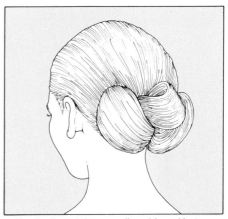

7. The final result is an easily achieved but elaborate looking woven effect.

Plaits (braids)

Plaits (braids) never really go out of fashion because there are so many ways they can be worn. What is popular with one generation looks old-fashioned to another, which will be wearing plaits (braids) in an entirely different way. What is regarded as a school-girl image in one age is the height of chic in the next.

Plaiting (braiding) is the process of intertwining strands of hair – usually three strands – one over the other in a regular pattern to form one thick strand. More than three strands can be intertwined and the thickness of the final plait is governed by how much hair is taken up in each strand. Make sure that you use covered bands to secure the hair, so that the hair is in no danger of being damaged.

Variations of this technique are known as weaving or cornrowing, after the style of plaiting done with corn stalks in farming communities at harvest time to make goodluck charms. Some astonishing effects can be achieved with weaving, and skilled hairdressers have made an art of dressing long hair into shapes that simulate hats with picture brims, boaters or jockey caps. Usually the hair is

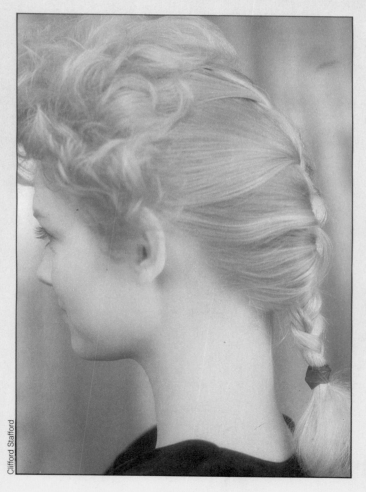

Clifford Stafford

CORNWEAVING YOUR HAIR

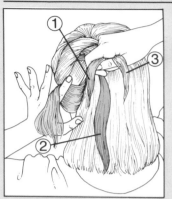

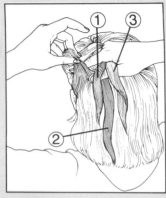

1. Take 3 sections of the hair, all of equal quantity (shown as **1,2,3,** in pictures). Start to plait (braid) the hair as you would normally; one section in turn over the other.

2. Take a new section of the hair from the left side of your head and add it to section **1**.

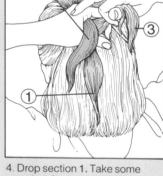

3. Take section **2**, which has been hanging down the middle of your plait and plait it into the hair as normal.

4. Drop section **1**. Take some extra hair from the right side of your head and add it to section **3**, as you did for section **1**. The sections must be clearly defined before they join the plait.

5. Repeat, until you have reached the nape of your neck. You will have collected all your hair from the right and left sides of your head, alternately.

Plaits (braids) have come a long way from their school-girl image with styles like this. The mood is young, but the look is sophisticated, with the perfect balance of frothy curls, neatly swept-back sides and pert pigtail.

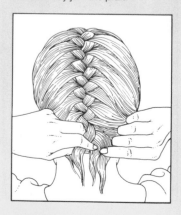

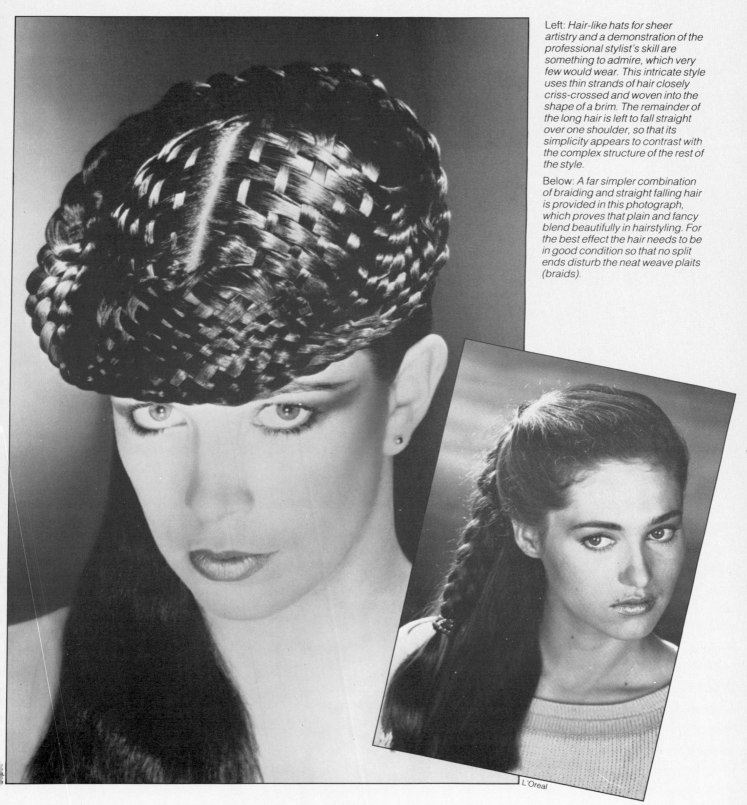

Left: *Hair-like hats for sheer artistry and a demonstration of the professional stylist's skill are something to admire, which very few would wear. This intricate style uses thin strands of hair closely criss-crossed and woven into the shape of a brim. The remainder of the long hair is left to fall straight over one shoulder, so that its simplicity appears to contrast with the complex structure of the rest of the style.*

Below: *A far simpler combination of braiding and straight falling hair is provided in this photograph, which proves that plain and fancy blend beautifully in hairstyling. For the best effect the hair needs to be in good condition so that no split ends disturb the neat weave plaits (braids).*

L'Oreal

woven over a shaped piece of card to achieve these stunning effects.

A recent fashion in plaiting called for dozens of very slim plaits, interwoven with tiny beads, forming the upper layer of the hair. It was inspired by traditional African styling techniques and was quickly taken up as 'the ethnic look' in America and Europe. Once the hair has been plaited in this elaborate and intricate style, the wearer will keep the style intact for several weeks, just confining shampooing to the roots of the hair and scalp to eliminate greasiness and leaving the fine plaits and beads untouched.

Plaiting is a convenient method of keeping long hair off the face and out of the way. Traditionally, it's a symmetrical style with two plaits, one each side of the head. A more fashionable look, especially popular with long-haired girls on holiday at beach resorts, is the single plait hanging down over the nape of the neck onto the back. It is an adaptation of the Chinaman's queue or sailor's pigtail and

ideal for keeping the hair neat while swimming and sunbathing.

Plaits do not have to hang straight down from the head. Often a single plait is coiled round and pinned at the nape of the neck in a style known as a plaited chignon, or plaits are coiled on each side of the head in what is called the earphones style, which had its heyday in the 1920s. Softer, more flowing, variations on this theme are still part of modern day styling techniques.

There are any number of variations on the plaiting (braiding) theme. The one major requirement is that the hair should be long enough to catch into plaits and cut to all one length rather than be layered, which would not be suitable as it would create a wispy, untidy effect with odd lengths of hair sticking out from various parts of the plait. For the neatest effect it is worth slightly dampening the hair with water as you plait or using a little hairspray or styling gel to keep the strands smooth and even for a polished-looking effect.

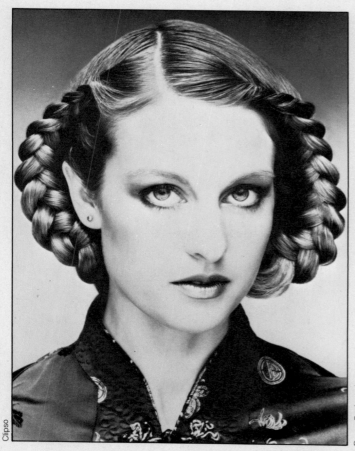

Clipso

Above: *This modern-day version of 'earphones' takes thick plaits (braids) around the head and* *anchors them at the back instead of the sides of the head.*

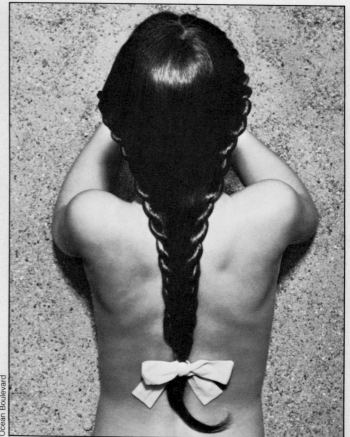

Ocean Boulevard

Above: *A wonderful way with long hair at holiday time is 'the plait'. One thick braid down the back* *can be changed into a sophisticated style with side weaving.*

The history of hair accessories

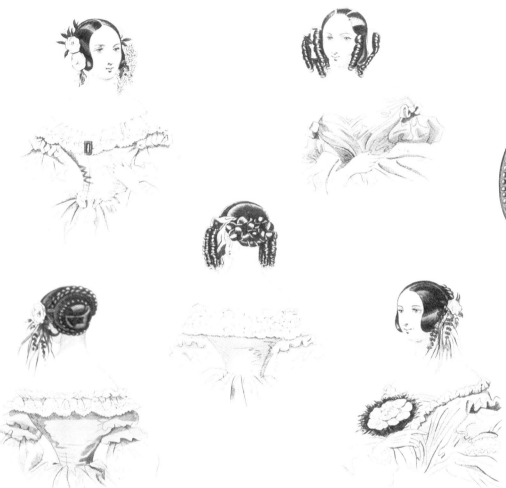

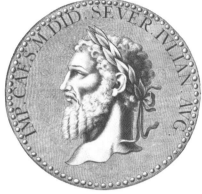

The victorious laurel leaf wreath worn by Roman emperors must surely have been the forerunner to the plaited (braided) hairstyle. Decorated with a ribbon tie it looks like a version of the plaited be-ribboned styles of early Victorian times, shown here.

Here is the same ornate theme, with the plaits supplemented by ringlets and curls, leaves, flowers and fruits to create a variety of looks that owe more to accessories than to the actual hairstyle which remains pretty constant throughout.

The history of hair accessories is as old as humanity. It is quite probable that women in the Stone Age made use of little pieces of animal bone to tame their hair. Then, of course, fashion, as such, did not exist and the use of the bones would have been for purely practical reasons.

We know the Egyptians, Greeks, Romans and Chinese wore hair accessories because examples of such have been found in burial tombs and ancient carvings and statues indicate that hair ornaments were worn. They could have been symbolic – think of the laurel wreath that went to the victor or the fine gold circlets worn by Roman women to indicate wealth or status – or they could have been solely for ornamentation.

In Anglo-Saxon times in Britain, head-tires, or circlets of gold set with jewels, were worn by women to denote rank, and veils were held in place over the head with elaborately carved bone pins. By Norman times, hair ornamentation had become an established part of life when women started interlacing their plaits (braids) with ribbons. Because extreme length in plaits was admired, they increased the illusion of length by encasing the ends of the plaits in silk tubes with ornamental tassels or by attaching metal cylinders to the very tips.

Hair ornamentation continued to increase, becoming grander and more elaborate all the time to signify the difference between the leisured rich and the working classes. During the reign of Louis XVI and Marie Antoinette in France in the latter part of the eighteenth century, hairstyles sported yards of lace and ribbons and were built up so high, stretched over wire frames, that they brushed against chandeliers and made it necessary for doors to be rebuilt for more headroom.

After that period a little more sense prevailed and hair ornamentation became simpler until, finally, it became just decoration for decoration's sake rather than a way of denoting class and status.

Accessories for today

Hair ornaments and accessories are becoming increasingly popular today to complement hair cuts and hair colouring. There are a wide variety of accessories available to choose from. They can be fun to wear and can transform a rather mundane hairstyle into a dramatic and original creation.

Almost any hair type can benefit, so whether your hair is short or long, straight or curly, fine or thick, you can choose and use any of the many thousands of accessories on sale today – and let fashion go to your head.

Whether the accessories comprise plastic bulldog clips (butterfly clips) or butterfly-shaped feathers, a classic rose or hairslide (barrette), there is always something to put in the hair.

Accessories have the same advantage as pieces of jewelry of making you stand out and acting as a trademark to your style and personality. They are often worn as an evening fashion to give a slightly more elaborate style to go with more dressy clothes worn to parties and the theatre. And if you like wearing hair accessories there certainly is no shortage of choice.

Styles featuring accessories

Fashions come and fashions go in hair accessories as much as in clothes and jewelry, mainly because hair accessories follow the same trends that dictate what we are going to wear this season or next.

Hair accessories are usually influenced by styling looks created by media personalities, pop stars and actresses. Some styles have to feature accessories, if only to achieve or maintain the style. A prime example is the ponytail and, as most people soon discover, rubber bands are difficult to put on and take off again without removing quite a few strands of hair with them. So the answer is a rubber band covered in thread or fabric,

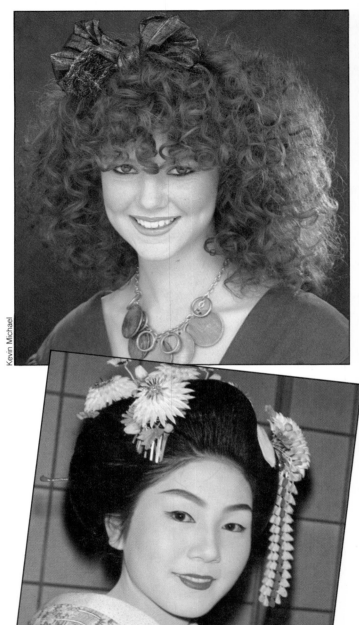

Kevin Michael

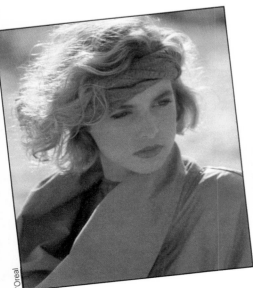

L'Oreal

Top right: *An extravagant bow is still one of the easiest ways to dress up a wash-and-wear hairstyle.*

Left: *Scarves are versatile accessories. They can give an outdoor look ideal for the country, or a sophisticated evening look.*

Above: *Traditional Eastern costumes call for the type of highly elaborate hair decoration which is now fashionable in the West.*

Right: *Brightly coloured, crownless hats are ideal for shading the eyes and keeping the sun off delicate skin without flattening the hair.*

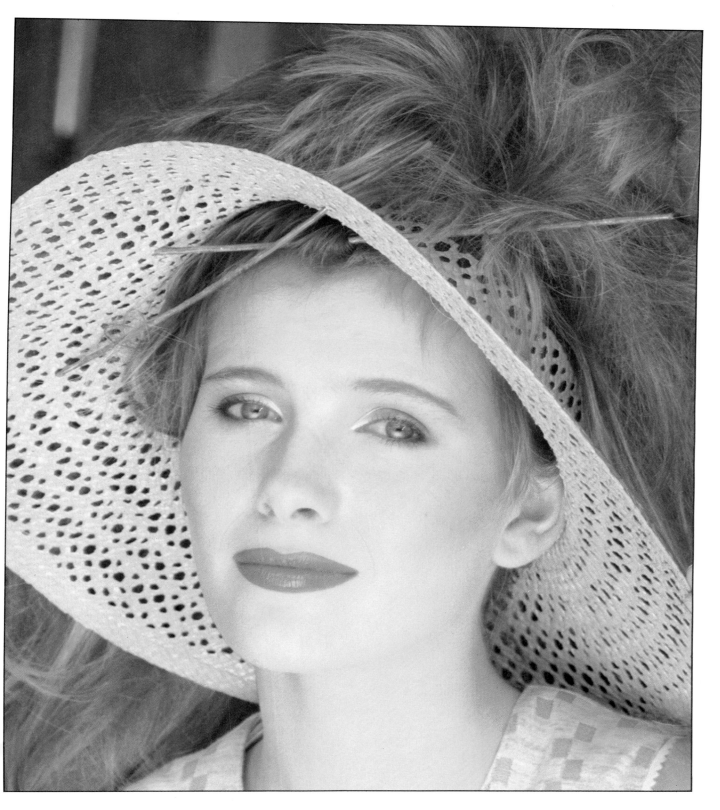

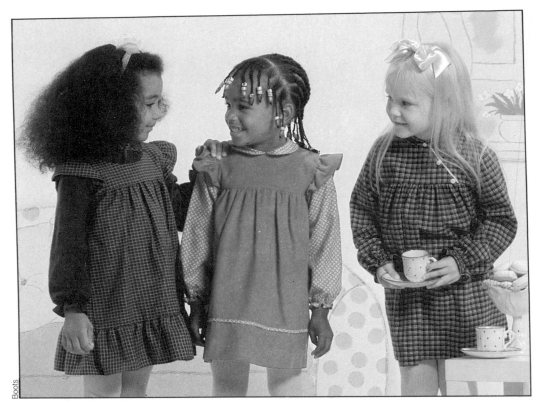

Girls love to dress up, so what better way than letting them experiment and play with hair accessories. Alice bands, ribbons, headbands and bows are generally fairly inexpensive to buy and, as well as being fun to wear, can serve a useful purpose in encouraging young people towards good grooming and developing a fashion sense.

They serve another purpose, too. They help keep the hair neat, stop it blowing about and getting into tangles which can be damaging as well as being painful to comb out. However, be sure that the accessories you buy are suitable for young children and that they have no sharp teeth or rough edges that could tear at the hair.

which still has the stretchiness but not the hair-damaging properties of rubber bands without covering.

Often a fashion for a hair accessory is created by a hairdresser who uses some fairly simple, pedestrian object as a way of drawing attention to his work. If a photograph of the hairstyle appears in a magazine, and especially if the magazine is a glossy and authoritative fashion source, the idea will swiftly catch on and a hair accessories manufacturer will be quick to jump on the bandwagon with a version of the original object meant especially for dressing up the hair.

An example of this was the chopstick look, developed in a London salon as part of a perming process. The stylist thought the long sticks used as perming rods looked good in the hair and used them in his next styling session with a magazine, on a dark-haired model sporting a Japanese-influenced hairstyle.

Types of accessories

Fancy combs are always popular and, with modern-day plastics which can easily simulate tortoiseshell and horn, the designs are as often as not based on the kinds of styles worn at the turn of the century. Worn to clip hair back from the sides of the face, they are not very good in fine hair as they tend to slip and slither out of place too easily. They can look particularly effective, however, in thick, heavy hairstyles.

Another craze has been for bulldog clips (butterfly clips), said to have originated on an Italian beach where girls used the office variety to keep hair from trailing in the water. Hair accessory manufacturers quickly caught on to this vogue and turned out replicas of the clips in bright-coloured plastic. They are very similar to the wave-setting clips that were much in use in the 1930s. So with hair accessories, almost anything can be tried.

As a group, girls tend to wear more hair accessories than any other. Ribbons and bows are favoured by young girls and fine hair that is limp and fly-away needs to be kept in place with the use of slides (barrettes) and hairclips (bobby pins).

Saving money

Accessories need not be at all expensive. Brightly coloured plastic slides and combs may be very cheap and cheerful. You probably already have in your wardrobe a choice of silk or cotton scarves you can wind through your hair or wrap round your head. Hair ribbons cost very little to buy – and may not cost you anything. You can, for example, make do with those shiny gift wrap bows you use to decorate Christmas parcels.

Switches and hairpieces

The main centre of the hairpiece market is the Far East. Originally the fashion market grew up in Hong Kong because Asian hair was readily available for use in the manufacture of switches and hairpieces. There was no shortage of women ready to sell their long straight hair. Moreover, Asian hair was strong enough to withstand the bleaching, colouring and perming necessary for making it match with European hair.

Also there was the cheap labour in Hong Kong and, in the mid 1960s, hundreds of one-room factories sprung up in shanty-towns all over the island. By the beginning of the 1970s hairpieces, switches and natural hair had become one of Hong Kong's fastest growing exports. But rocketing world demand was already depleting the supplies of natural hair, and synthetic fibres had to be developed to supplement this resource.

The earliest synthetic fibre hairpieces were made from nylon blends and were not very successful. Apart from being extremely difficult to manage, because of attracting static which created the problem of fly-away hair, these hairpieces had an unnatural gloss. They were followed by acrylic fibres, which looked and felt a little better, and then by modacrylics.

Other fibres have followed, including one called Elura which has a cuticle-like surface bringing it closer to the look and feel of natural hair. They are washable: just use a mild shampoo and plenty of lukewarm water to rinse all traces of lather from the hairpiece, and comb well with a bone or metal comb which avoids creating static.

Hairpieces usually come on a circular open-weave base, and in a variety of shapes and sizes. For example, the half-head hairpiece (wiglet) that is usually set on an Alice (head) band or comb that fixes it to the hair across the crown, adding height to a style, or padding out thinning hair, or the long slim strand, set on a small round base, which is ideal for twisting into a chignon or bun at the nape or top of the head. Your hairdresser can teach you an infinite variety of possible hairstyles. Many models have learned the tricks of such instant transformation, using a seemingly endless number of hair accessories, from plaits (braids) to chignons. If you take hairpieces seriously, allow plenty of time for choosing them and don't be afraid to ask about cleaning and after-care.

In all cases it is necessary to match the piece as exactly as possible to your own hair colouring, unless you are going frankly fake and adding a constrasting coloured plait or colourful bunch of curls to your style. When fixing a hairpiece on the head it usually needs to be blended in with your natural hair and coiled or curled into place and fixed with hairpins (bobby pins).

Hairpieces made of synthetic fibres are usually quite cheap. However, if they are made using real hair, carefully colour matched to your own, it does of course, make them quite expensive.

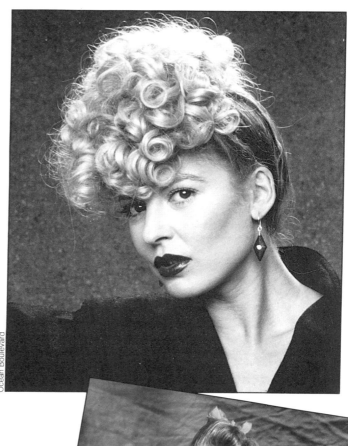

Ocean Boulevard

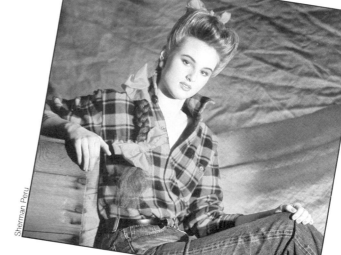

Sherman Peru

Above: *Turn short hair into long hair with a hairpiece. A topknot can provide an instant transformation with a tumble of curls anchored in place, while the natural hair is smoothed back or pinned securely under the piece.*

Below: *A hair extension, pinned at the root and woven through your own hair, decorates the top or back of the head, falling midway between being a hairpiece and a hair ornament. It can be made with false hair, fabric and feathers.*

Party time

Use a change of hairstyle as part of dressing up for a party. This gives you plenty of scope for choosing the kind of zany, fun style you would not contemplate for everyday wear and the opportunity to sport crazy accessories that would never go with your workday clothes.

Parties are meant to be fun. They are often held as a celebration, sometimes in fancy dress and sometimes to follow a set theme. They give you the chance to try out a new look – a new way of wearing your hair – so take advantage of them and dare to be different.

Make the most of your hair with some elaborate styling techniques that will make others turn their heads to look at yours. You can call on hairpieces and hair accessories, any manner of baubles, spangles and beads, to dress up your hair in any way you choose. You can use gels and mousses to contour your hair into different shapes. You can spray all over with glitter for colourful effects and be as outrageous as you like. Wear fresh flowers in your hair for a pretty and feminine effect. Weave tiny, brightly coloured nylon plaits (braids) or ribbons through the hair for a youthful style. Add a touch of drama with a sleeked back style held in place with a black velvet bow, or fabric rolls that fall half way between a hat and hair accessory. The possibilities are endless and governed only by your imagination and personal taste.

There is one important thing to remember, though. You want to feel comfortable throughout your evening out and confident that your hairstyle will stay in place, so arm yourself with spare hairpins, grips and clips and take along a small can of hairspray or tube of mousse, so you can easily touch up or re-anchor a slipping style to see you through the party.

Clipso

PUTTING IN PLAITS

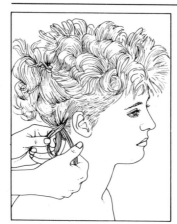

1. Start by taking a 1-inch (2.5 centimetre) square of hair behind the ear and plaiting it to the end of the length of hair.

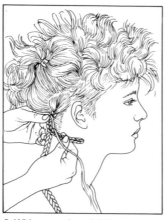

2. With extension plait in one hand carefully pull the natural plaited hair through the loop at the top end of the extension plait.

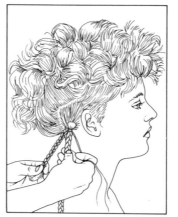

3. Take a length of wool and wind it from the root of the natural hair to a couple of inches below the join, and secure.

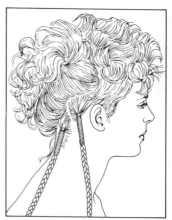

4. Once you have secured the extension plait, you can be assured that it will stay in place for as long as you want.

Pretty party styles rely a lot on buttons, bows and braids. They can be highly ornamented, like the style on the left which has a mass of coloured ribbons and strips of fabric threaded through and wrapped round the hair. Or they can be altogether simpler, like the style on the right, relying on just a twist of coloured braiding to contrast with the colour of the hair or match the shade of the dress.

They can be like the style below, which incorporates several tiny strands of brightly coloured false hair, fixed with pins close to the scalp, and long thin braids cascading down each side.

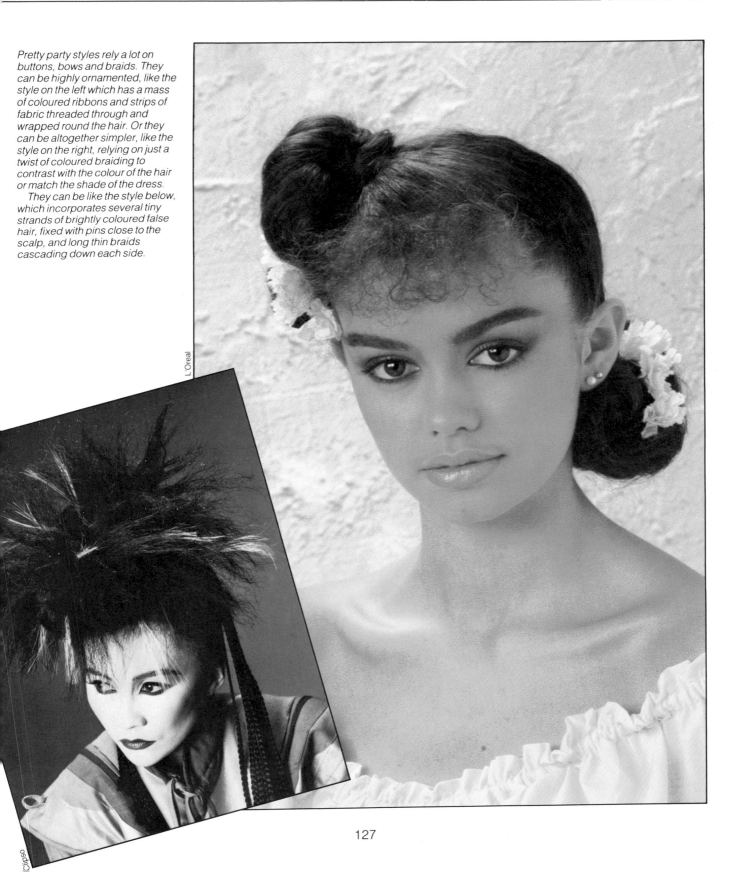

L'Oréal

Clipso

127

Sophisticated hair

How do you give everyday hair the glamorous evening look? The answer is: practice usually makes perfect, even if initially you may have to ask your hairdresser for help and advice. A perm, for example, could add interesting texture to very straight hair, especially when it is short and therefore limited in possibilities.

When the hair is long, and you plan to wear it in a sophisticated chignon for that special evening, your hairdresser could show you how to achieve a softening, feminine effect with tendrils. Tendrils can look untidy if you just pull them out of your hair. They are much prettier when you crimp them. This means taking a small section of hair and plaiting (braiding) it tightly while it is wet. Once the hair is dry, the plaits (braids) are unwound and the crimped hair is allowed to hang full-length.

A chignon, also known as a bun, can be placed virtually anywhere on the head. The hair can be gathered at the back of the head and twisted to be fastened lengthwise along the scalp. To be secure, it needs to be fastened along its entire length, preferably with hairpins. Take your time to practise this style.

Try wearing the style one evening, when it doesn't matter. You can then discover just how long it will stay up and remain in shape. If you have just washed your hair, it may be best not to use conditioner which can make the hair rather slippery.

Earrings can give focus and enhance your hair style and facial features. If you intend to use them, show them to your stylist or try them when you have your dress rehearsal.

Clipso

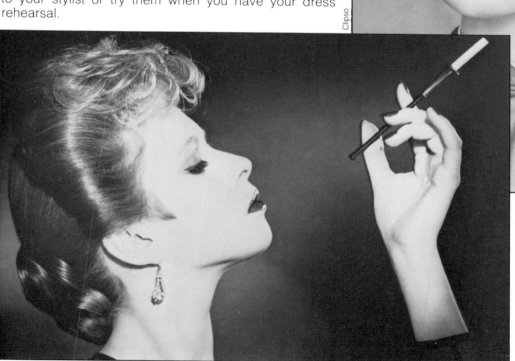

Clifford Stafford

Sophisticated evenings call for sophisticated hairstyles, which rely more on clever hairdressing techniques than on fun accessories. The style on the left combines chignon curls and tousled fringe curls for its good looks, while the style above has a carefully sleeked fringe (bangs) contrasting with the crimped tendrils at the temple. Opposite is an example of elegant braiding that dresses the hair up to complement an ornate neckline.

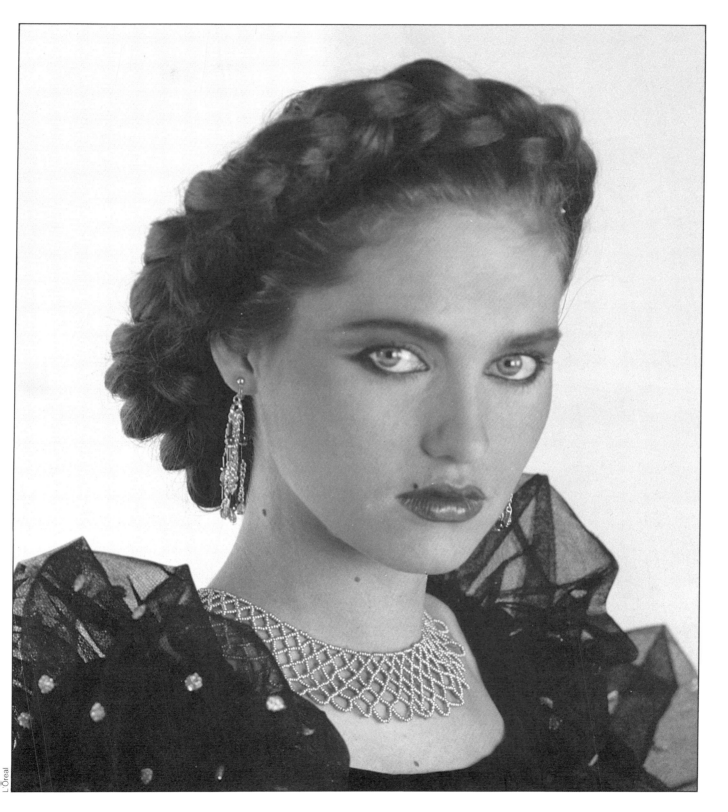

Styling with glasses

Glasses have become a major fashion accessory and many men and women take advantage of this fact with a whole wardrobe of well-designed frames that suit different outfits and the different occasions for which they are worn.

In every case, the tops of the frames should line up with your eyebrows. If they don't, you will have two sets of lines and this is most unflattering. Whatever type of glasses you choose they should fit comfortably. This means that they must sit firmly on the nose and cling to the head without feeling too tight.

By matching frames not only to clothes but also to hairstyles and face shape combined, you can create a more flattering or striking look.

Hairstyle

When you wear glasses it is all too easy for them to dominate your face, rather than for them to form part of your overall look and you can solve the problem, if this is what has happened to you, with a change of hairstyle. The length of your hair and the shape in which it is styled can

provide a balance to spectacle frames and show them off.

A general rule is that you should keep hair away from the temples and also avoid too heavy a fringe that will 'fight' with the top of the spectacle frame. With bold, square-shaped frames, it is often good to have a softening curly face-framing style. Light-coloured, metal frames tend to go better with fair rather than dark hair, whereas heavy, dark frames can be overpowering if your hair is blond or grey.

This is an aspect men quite often overlook. Unlike women, they are not used to working out colour harmony in make-up and have only the vaguest idea of what suits them, especially from the point of view of colour.

Upswept styles remain constantly popular with older women and certainly have a more flattering line for mature faces which benefit from the lift this shape of frame gives.

Face shape

Provided you have chosen your spectacle frames carefully to suit the shape of your face, and your existing style is right for you, there should be no need for a drastic

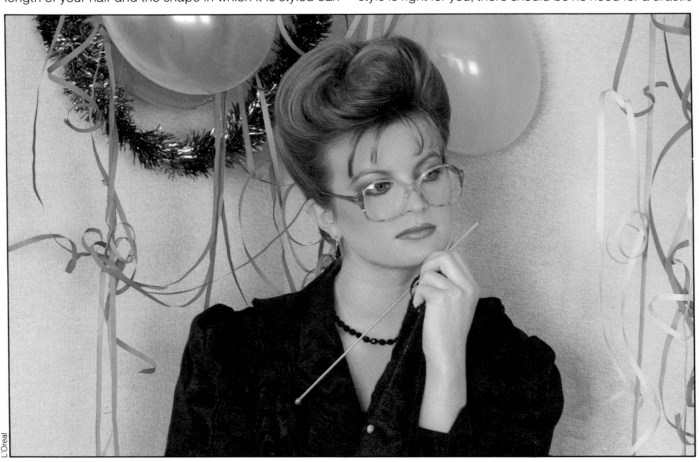

L'Oreal

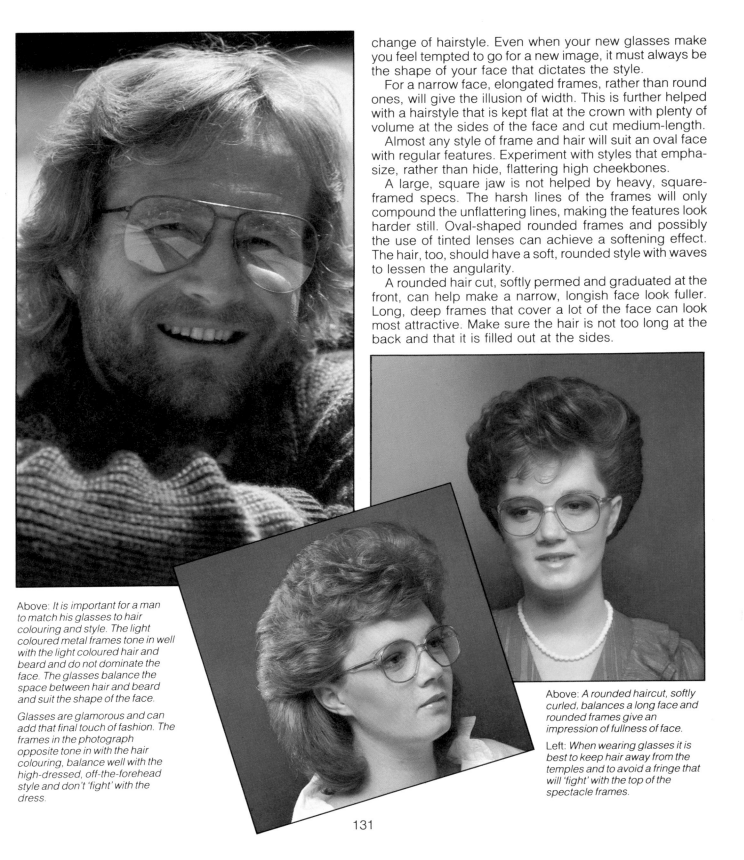

change of hairstyle. Even when your new glasses make you feel tempted to go for a new image, it must always be the shape of your face that dictates the style.

For a narrow face, elongated frames, rather than round ones, will give the illusion of width. This is further helped with a hairstyle that is kept flat at the crown with plenty of volume at the sides of the face and cut medium-length.

Almost any style of frame and hair will suit an oval face with regular features. Experiment with styles that emphasize, rather than hide, flattering high cheekbones.

A large, square jaw is not helped by heavy, square-framed specs. The harsh lines of the frames will only compound the unflattering lines, making the features look harder still. Oval-shaped rounded frames and possibly the use of tinted lenses can achieve a softening effect. The hair, too, should have a soft, rounded style with waves to lessen the angularity.

A rounded hair cut, softly permed and graduated at the front, can help make a narrow, longish face look fuller. Long, deep frames that cover a lot of the face can look most attractive. Make sure the hair is not too long at the back and that it is filled out at the sides.

Above: *It is important for a man to match his glasses to hair colouring and style. The light coloured metal frames tone in well with the light coloured hair and beard and do not dominate the face. The glasses balance the space between hair and beard and suit the shape of the face.*

Glasses are glamorous and can add that final touch of fashion. The frames in the photograph opposite tone in with the hair colouring, balance well with the high-dressed, off-the-forehead style and don't 'fight' with the dress.

Above: *A rounded haircut, softly curled, balances a long face and rounded frames give an impression of fullness of face.*

Left: *When wearing glasses it is best to keep hair away from the temples and to avoid a fringe that will 'fight' with the top of the spectacle frames.*

Styling with hats

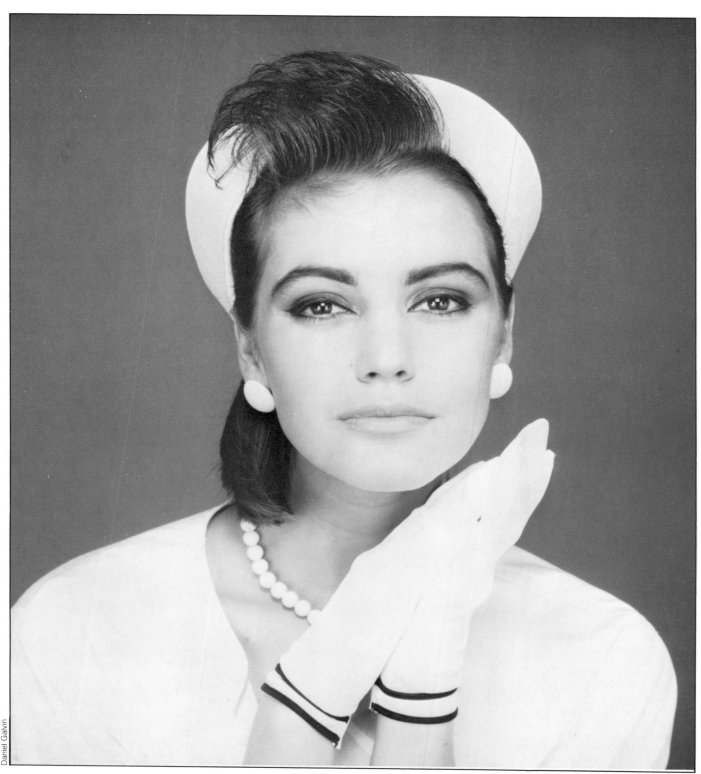

Daniel Galvin

Above: *Hair and hat in perfect harmony for a picture of fashion.*

132

There must be just about as many styles in hats as there are in hair fashions. And, like hairstyles, you need to choose them to suit your face and make-up, as part of a fashion ensemble and to meet the demands of different occasions.

A scruffy hairstyle will take away from the look of a hat, so it is obvious that hat and hairstyle should flow in one harmonious line. It will be up to you to decide whether your hair looks best completely tucked away under the hat or showing curls around the brim.

However, there are some general guidelines for co-ordinating definite styles of hats with particular hairstyles. Hats that are severe or masculine call for a softening effect to offset them, so a trilby (fedora) style will look good when worn with hair that is styled in a plait (braid) or in ringlet curls that add a feminine touch to the whole look. A glamorous style, such as a wide-brimmed picture hat, looks its best when the hair is worn in a sleek, smooth style that does not detract from its elegant lines.

Conversely, a saucy matelot style hat with a turned-up brim or a beret usually benefit from a froth of curls beneath, and a demure-looking straw boater looks great when it is offset by a long, straight 'little-girl' hairstyle. The tiny pillbox won't benefit from being swamped by a mass of flowing curls but will look far better on a close-to-the-head hairstyle.

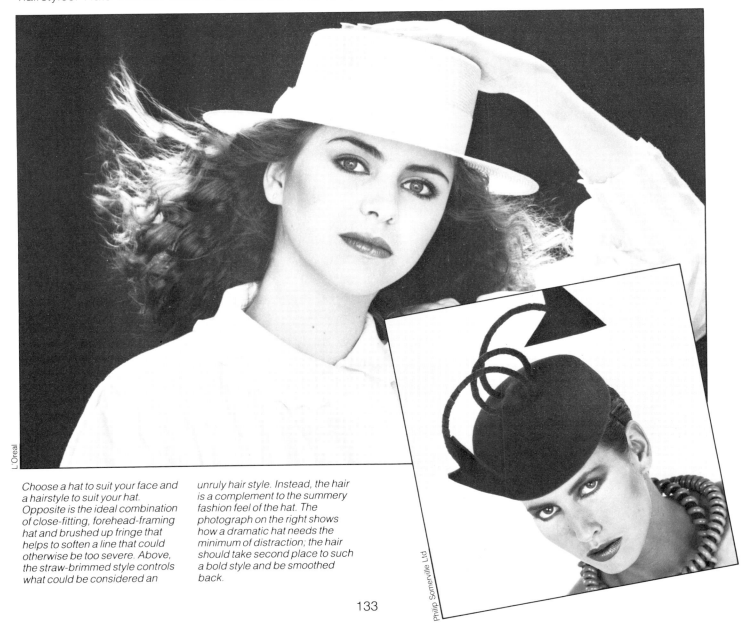

L'Oreal

Philip Somerville Ltd

Choose a hat to suit your face and a hairstyle to suit your hat. Opposite is the ideal combination of close-fitting, forehead-framing hat and brushed up fringe that helps to soften a line that could otherwise be too severe. Above, the straw-brimmed style controls what could be considered an unruly hair style. Instead, the hair is a complement to the summery fashion feel of the hat. The photograph on the right shows how a dramatic hat needs the minimum of distraction; the hair should take second place to such a bold style and be smoothed back.

133

Hairstyles fit for a bride will take into consideration the veil that she will wear for her walk down the aisle. Most important, though, is that the front hairline should be as neat as possible so it will not be too disturbed when the bride sweeps the veil off her face after the ceremony.

Either choose a style that is smoothed back from the hairline, with wispy corkscrew curls to soften the line, or choose one that is dressed in smooth rolls off the face. Both achieve the necessary neat front hairline.

As a general rule, long hair tends to suit veils better than short hair and it looks its best if left to hang loose, following the line of the veil, rather than dressed up on the crown.

Whether the veil is classic, Victorian or modern will also have an influence on how the hairstyle it sits on is dressed.

Not all brides wear a veil. Of course, for some, the choice is just a simple headress and in many ways this means that the hairstyle is even more crucial. As the bride spends a great deal of time with her back to the congregation, obviously it is the back of the hairstyle which assumes importance.

Finally, don't forget that your hairstyle must also cope with the honeymoon. No matter how elaborate it is for the wedding day, it should give you the option to turn it overnight into a pretty wash-and-wear style that can be kept in shape with the flick of a brush.

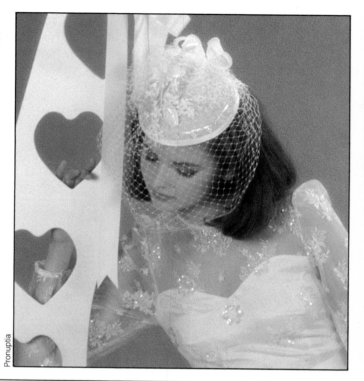

Pronuptia

MAKING SURE YOUR HAIR LOOKS GOOD

For your hair to look good on your wedding day, you need a little careful planning at least six to eight weeks before 'the day'.

○ Out-of-condition hair needs taking care of with a series of regular conditioning treatments over a period of at least two months - either at a hairdressing salon or with good treatment products at home.

○ Work out what kind of hairstyle will go best with your veil and have your hair cut well in advance of the wedding. This gives the hair time to settle down and you time to get used to coping with the style. Have a neatening-up trim a few days before the wedding.

○ If your hair relies on a permanent wave, have it done about a month before the wedding, to let the curl settle.

○ Practise fixing on the veil before the actual day, so

there is no danger of feeling it slip during the ceremony. Estimate what pins, clips (barrettes) or small combs sewn on to the veil you will need to keep it secure.

○ Allow plenty of time on the wedding day to have your hair shampooed, set and styled. If it is to be professionally done, book an appointment well in advance to avoid last-minute hitches.

○ Preferably, have the stylist come to you at home - most salons will do this for an extra fee to cover travelling time - to save yourself time and allow you to cope with doing your nails (*hands* are important, as they are on show while putting on rings, signing the register, cutting the cake etc) or getting on with your make-up while your hair dries.

○ Use a good setting lotion or plenty of hairspray to ensure your style holds well throughout the ceremony and the reception.

As the bride you are the centre of attention on your wedding day, so make sure that your "crowning glory" does you justice. Your hair should be in tip-top condition.

Be sure that your hairstyle suits the accessories you choose for your hair, whether you are planning to wear a veil, or hat or a

simple posy of flowers. If you do intend to wear an ornament of some sort in your hair make sure that it will be secure and comfortable during the whole ceremony, since the last thing you will want to be worrying about is the threat of a slipping hairdo.

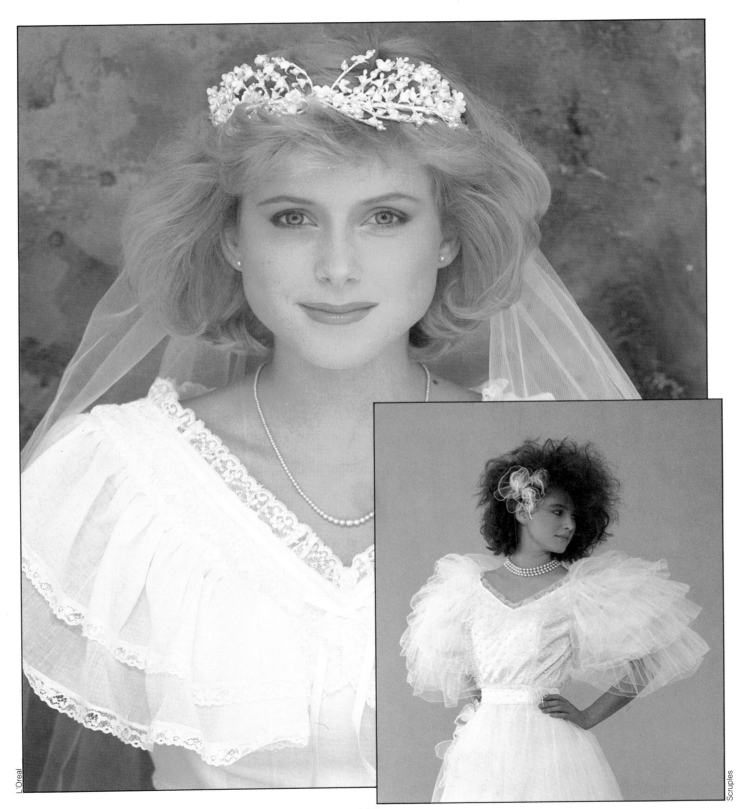

L'Oreal

Scruples

Fashion wigs

Fashion wigs made today are a far cry from the heavy cap styles mass-produced in the 1960s, which was the decade of the heyday of wigs. They are now ultra lightweight, and are positioned on lace bases that are airy, cool and comfortable to wear.

Fun and fashion wigs often come in crazy colours and are cut into exaggerated stepped shapes. They also come in natural-looking hair colours and offer you a chance of suddenly appearing with long hair in place of your naturally short crop. Fashion wigs are easy to put on, comfortable, and, if they have been well cut and shaped especially to suit you, it is hard to tell that they really are wigs and not your own hair.

You can usually buy a fashion wig, take it out of its box or bag and simply brush it into shape. However, skilled hairdressers can probably help in making the same wig look a lot more natural and suited to your face. They can alter the face shape by thinning or trimming the hair. Although they will not be able to perm a fibre or Asian hair wig, they can still re-style it with a certain amount of back-brushing. Hairdressers can also cut fringes (bangs) to camouflage a receding hairline or brush the hair off the sides of the face to produce a bright wide-eyed effect. On the other hand, they can brush the hair forward on to the face to make a square chin look more delicate.

To put a wig on you first need to pin down your own hair, in flat curls against the scalp. Then fit on the wig at the front, holding it firmly against the forehead while you ease it down at the back and sides. Next, adjust the fit, which should be firm but not tight, securing the wig if necessary with a hairpin or two at the crown.

Unless the wig has a fringe (bangs), it is worth teasing out a bit of your own hair at the front and blending it in with the wig, for a more natural look — that is, if you have chosen a wig that is the same colour as your own hair.

However, no matter how light and airy the base of a wig is, it is still rather like wearing a close-fitting cap — especially with a full head of hair — and this will make the scalp feel rather hot. This can cause sweating and encourage the glands to over-activate which, in turn can lead to irritation of the scalp.

Because of the heat, sweating and extra greasiness, it is important that you keep both your scalp and wig scrupulously clean and carefully wash them both very frequently.

Half wigs (wiglets)

Half wigs are good for bolstering up hair that is naturally thin, for dressing up a glamorous evening style, and for making a quick change from day to evening wear. They come in a variety of shapes and sizes such as the half-head hairpiece that is usually set on an Alice (head) band.

It is always necessary to match the piece as exactly as possible to your own hair colouring, unless you are going frankly fake and adding a contrasting coloured plait (braid) or colourful bunch of curls to your style. When fixing a hairpiece on the head it usually needs to be blended in with your natural hair and coiled or curled into place and then fixed with hairpins (bobby pins).

Half wigs (wiglets) come in a choice of synthetic fibres, many of which are quite cheap, or they can be made up of real hair carefully colour matched to your own. This does, of course, make them quite expensive.

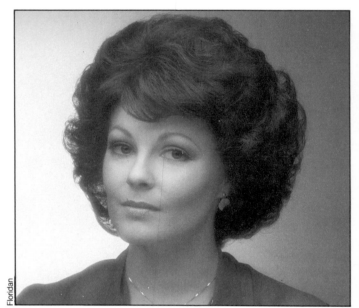

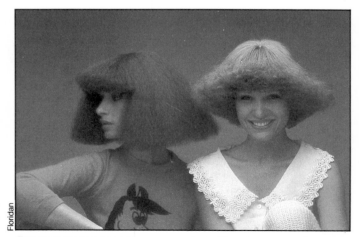

Fashion wigs can provide countless possibilities for changing your style. They can be cut and coloured, so that you can look either demure or outrageous. Treat the wigs as if they were your own hair, keeping them in good condition all the time.

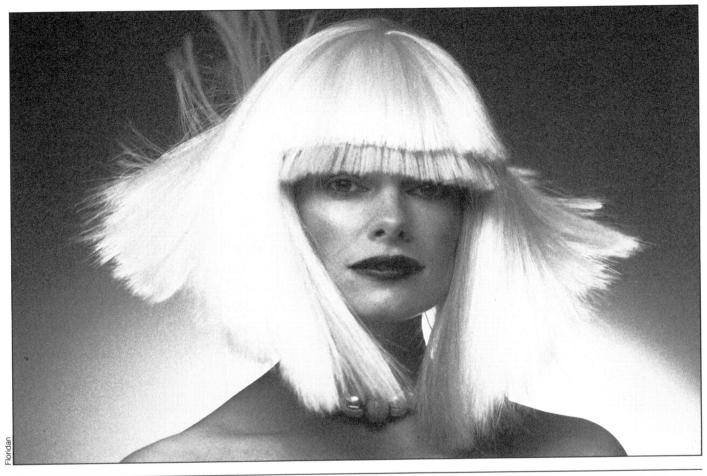

Floridan

STEP-BY-STEP PUTTING ON A WIG

STEP-BY-STEP PUTTING ON A WIG

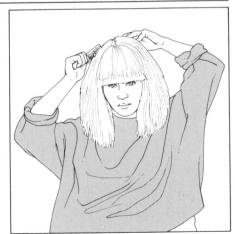

1. First secure your own hair into a flat bun or pleat or pin your curls away from the hair line.

2. Holding the wig at the back, with head angled down, position the front of the wig on the forehead and ease the wig over your own hair until it is in place.

3. Grip the base of the wig to your own hair with pins or curler grips on both sides, below the crown and at the nape. Then brush wig into style.

137

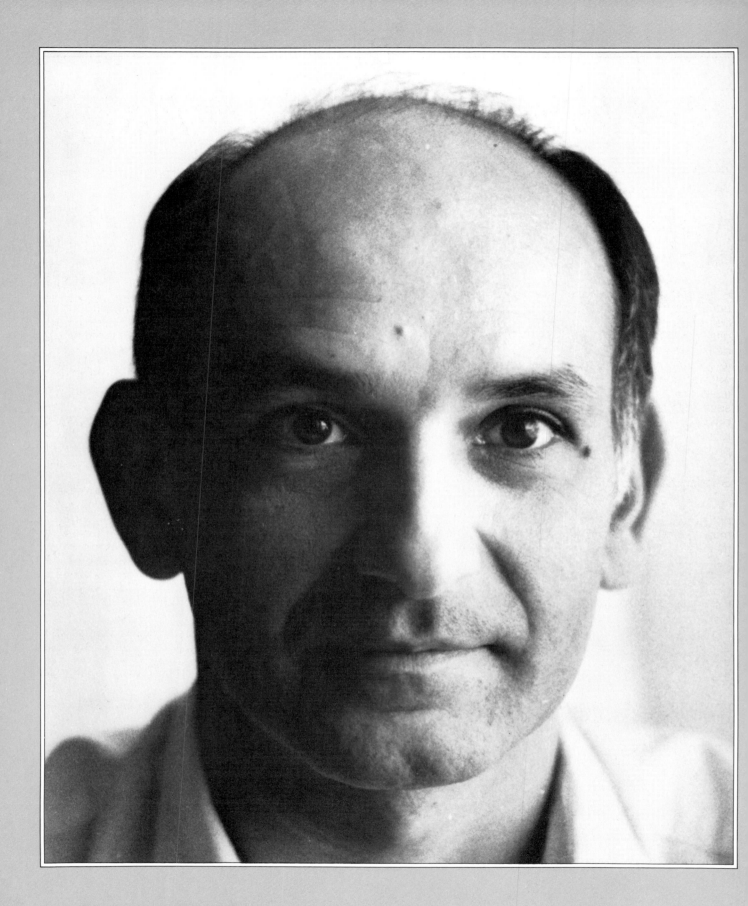

9
Thinning hair and hair loss

A seemingly endless number of causes have been attributed to baldness, including diet, stress, hormones, pollution and medication. The truth is that it is extremely difficult, if not impossible, at times to pinpoint one single, definite reason for baldness other than that the tendency to go bald is often hereditary. Our life-styles, so fraught with tensions and worries, are only partly to blame. But there seem to be just as many men living in primitive societies, away from pollution and pressures, who go bald just the same. The problem does not appear to be related to climate, either: baldness in men is just as prevalent in hot as it is in cold countries.

Sudden hair loss

Once in a while, almost everyone experiences a noticeable degree of hair falling out and this condition may continue for days and sometimes weeks. In the vast majority of cases, there is usually no cause for alarm. The hair loss is likely to be only temporary.

When sudden hair loss occurs, a trichologist will look closely at the scalp. Usually, a great many very short hairs will be visible. By examining the hair, the reasons for hair loss can often be identified. The ends of the hair provide the clue. If they taper to a point, it means the hairs are new and just emerging from the follicle. When the hair end is frayed or blunt, the hair has simply broken off very close to the scalp.

When the hair has temporarily fallen out, it can be a symptom of a recent illness, an emotional trauma, or both. Other reasons include drugs, a hormonal imbalance, poor diet, vitamin deficiency – particularly in the B and C vitamins – and sometimes also a deficiency of minerals such as zinc, iron and sulphur. We do not yet know or understand fully why hair loss sometimes occurs on what appears to be a healthy scalp, but what we do know is that it results from the hair follicles going into a prolonged period of rest.

Only about 80 per cent of our hair is growing – and it can last from about two to six years. The remaining 20 per cent of our hair is in the resting stage which lasts around three months before the hair is finally shed. After illness, childbirth, and often following emotional stress, a great many hairs enter this resting stage at the same time. Then, after a few months, all these hairs are shed more or less simultaneously, causing a far greater hair loss than is normal.

Hair loss can also be caused by traction, that is, pulling the hair too tight in a ponytail and using anything from rollers to slides (barrettes), fine-toothed combs and elastic bands. Once you have spotted the cause of this type of temporary hair loss, there is only one thing to do: stop! Throw out that hard brush and change that hairstyle, so you won't need to tie it back or use those damaging clips or bands.

If diet is the problem, take some vitamin and mineral supplements until you're feeling on top of the world again. Dietitians swear by brewer's yeast, taken after each meal, and Vitamin E, known as the anti-ageing vitamin, is said to be valuable in improving the circulation. Wheatgerm is also thought to be good for healthy, shining hair.

In about 400BC, Hippocrates – known as the 'father of medicine' – prescribed opium, mixed with rose or lily essence and made into an ointment with wine, acacia juice and olive oil, as a cure for thinning hair. Some 3400 years earlier, the mother of an Egyptian king recommended rubbing the head with a concoction of ground dogs' paws, dates and asses hooves cooked in oil. Other unappetizing cures included an application with a mixture made from burning live snakes – thought to be particularly restorative if the snakes were caught at full moon.

Although these weird mixtures are unlikely to have helped in themselves, we know today that massage of the scalp is both relaxing and restorative. Rather than a balm made of snakes, we now use high-frequency treatments with electrodes to stimulate and increase the blood circulation to the scalp. The means may be different, but the end result – with the beneficial effect on the blood circulation which stimulates the nerves and tiny blood vessels and forces them to distribute the essential nutrients to the papilla – is still very much the same.

How to style thinning hair

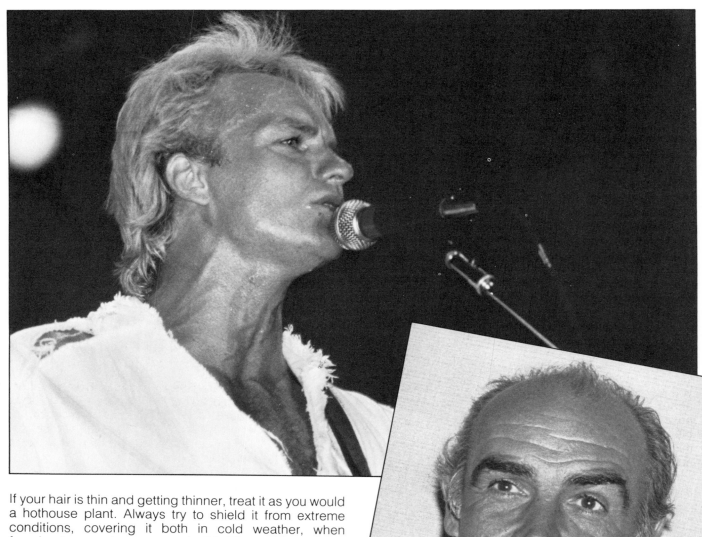

If your hair is thin and getting thinner, treat it as you would a hothouse plant. Always try to shield it from extreme conditions, covering it both in cold weather, when freezing temperatures can make it brittle, and in sunlight, which has a harsh, drying and bleaching effect. Avoid any drastic chemical styling methods such as perms or tints. Nature has given a warning that the hair is in a vulnerable state, so you had best heed it.

As we age, the growth of our hair gradually slows down and, as we turn grey, our hair goes through a process of decolouration, with pigment, air content and oil all involved, together with structural changes. After the menopause, the hair often becomes thinner through the metabolic changes that occur. Most women have little to worry about and complete hair loss at this time of life is very unlikely. Your hair will have been exposed to some rather harsh treatment over the years, so perhaps the time has come to give it a rest by giving it an easy-care face-flattering style that needs no strong chemicals or over-hot drying for setting.

For people in the public eye the problems of thinning hair can be difficult. Clever styling at the early stages of hair loss or wearing a toupee, can help to disguise the impending problem. Eventually, however, hair loss is something that you have to come to terms with. Sean Connery reached this stage with no apparent trauma and is as often seen with toupee as without.

With thinning hair, care is of the utmost importance. One way to start is to have a close look at the equipment you are using. Combs must not be too fine and bristle brushes should not have sharp tips that can scratch and damage the scalp. When combing the hair, never start at the scalp but always begin near the ends of the hair. Take your time and don't even try to comb or brush through the entire length in one go. Start at the ends and gradually move up, bit by bit. If you are tempted to back-comb your hair to give it a more bulky appearance, remember that a hairstyle has to be specially designed in order to be suitable for back-combing.

Avoid using curling tongs, (curling irons) electric rollers and blow dryers. Whenever possible, allow the hair to dry naturally, untangling it with the fingers before trying to comb it through. A conditioner can help protect the hair from external damage as well as giving it more shine and bounce. As it clings to the hair shaft, it will fill in the irregularities and make the hair smoother and easier to comb. Do not expect miracles from your conditioner, however, as it can only help the hair and does not affect the scalp.

A healthy scalp

Helping your scalp stay in a healthy condition means that you have to adopt a number of measures. Both internal and external factors are involved. Both are designed to ensure that the skin of the scalp is richly supplied by the blood circulation. In addition to an adequate, healthy diet, this can be achieved by helping the scalp to stay loose and relaxed with massage.

Use the tips of the fingers and rub the scalp well, avoiding any pull on the hair. Your hands should be used in a claw-like position, as though you were holding a round ball with the pads of the fingers only touching the scalp. Do not be afraid to apply a reasonable amount of pressure and let your fingers move in small, circular movements over the entire scalp. If you want to keep this massage going for some time, simply do it while resting your elbows on the table. You can even read a book while you're doing it, so that you will not get bored quickly. The longer you can keep it up, the better the results.

If the scalp is left for months or years without treatment, permanent thinning may result and the hair follicles could disappear altogether. This is why massage of the scalp is important in helping to improve the circulation.

Haircuts for thinning hair

Although it may be difficult to camouflage thinning hair, a top hairdresser can help you make the most of what you have left with a superb haircut. Thin, fine hair usually looks best if it is cut rather short so that the weight of the hair

does not flatten at the crown. What is known as a 'club cut' (blunt cut) in the trade will help the hair to keep its body.

Ideally, you should be able to cope with your hairstyle at home without any problems; a shake of the head should normally be enough for the hair to fall back in place.

If the hair is very fine and fly-away, a setting lotion can be useful at times. For extra body, blot the hair with an absorbent towel before applying the lotion.

Men whose hair is thinning can benefit from a short haircut. Cut really short, it will look much thicker. All the things women should do to keep their hair and scalp in good condition also apply to men. First and foremost, the hair must be kept scrupulously clean with good shampooing and conditioning treatments. A well-balanced diet, keep-fit programme and anything that can help control stress will be useful to help preserve the remaining hair.

Bald is beautiful!

It is a pity that so many men still equate hair loss with loss of sexual virility and strength and that this, in turn, is identified with ageing. Balding may indicate ageing because the death of the hair follicles is in fact a form of premature ageing. However, it only affects the scalp and not the body as a whole.

Women usually care little or nothing about whether a man has a full head of hair or not. Film stars, including Yul Brynner and Sean Connery, have proved this by remaining sex symbols to millions of women for decades. As far as women are concerned, when it comes to the opposite sex, bald really can be beautiful.

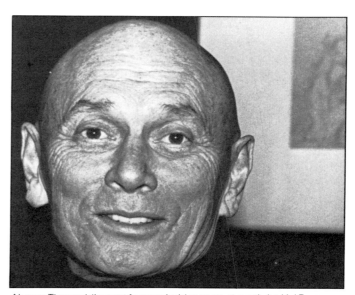

Above: *The world's most famous bald man must surely be Yul Brynner.*

Baldness in men, women and children

When someone loses hair on the head in patches, the first symptom is the sudden appearance of a white bald patch, usually round in shape. The surrounding hair may otherwise look quite healthy. The patch is usually about ½ an inch (1.2 centimetres) in diameter, matt white in appearance and may be surrounded by short hairs. If it is oval, this could mean that the baldness is spreading. It may spread with further patches and ultimately the patches could merge into a larger area. When total baldness occurs, the scalp is often as smooth and clean as a billiard ball.

Causes of thinning hair

As we get older, there is some wasting away of the tissues. As the shafts of the hairs become finer and shorter, the scalp will inevitably start to look as though it is only thinly covered with hairs.

Some illnesses and medical treatments often have hair loss as one of their unpleasant side-effects. Six to eight weeks after a high fever, it is quite common for the hair to fall out from every part of the scalp. This gives the trichologist a valuable clue: if the hair is gently pulled at the temples, and comes out in large tufts, the reason is probably a high, feverish illness some time previously.

Harsh perms, tints or bleaches may cause hair loss and even the use of a shampoo that is too alkaline. Rough treatment simply causes the hair to break and become brittle, reducing its elasticity.

Diffuse hair fall may be the result of skin diseases affecting the scalp, such as acute eczema or dermatitis. It can also be due to a fungal infection and, if this is the case, it is associated with a scaly scalp and broken hairs. When bald patches are caused by infectious skin diseases, an antibiotic is administered which circulates in the blood and is absorbed by the skin and hair follicles, destroying the infection. Ringworm in children can easily be mistaken for baldness, as one of its symptoms is a patch of inflammation with some scaling and hair loss. The patch gets larger and, when it stops growing, another patch appears elsewhere on the scalp. The scaly, inflamed areas may become infected with bacteria, producing a condition called impetigo. Impetigo can also be mistaken for baldness; the condition causes crusts to fall from the scalp. As the crusts fall, hairs entangled in the crusts also fall, producing a few small bald areas. These are slightly depressed and pink and do not enlarge. Fortunately, when the condition has cleared, the hairs usually grow in again very fast.

When there is diffuse hair loss without apparent infection of the scalp, the trichologist will have to pinpoint the reason. After a great nervous shock, it is quite common for all the hair to fall out about two weeks later. The hair growth usually resumes after one to three months.

When there is no local disease of the scalp and hair, the treatment aims at improving the circulation of the blood in the scalp. This means that every effort has to be made to improve the general state of health in the first place. In addition, drugs can be prescribed that are known to stimulate the hair follicles.

Baldness in men

For men going bald, one of the greatest temptations is to grow what remaining hair there is long to compensate for what is lacking on top of the head. This is a great mistake, as anybody would agree who has seen a cunningly grown and combed back lock that covers a bald pate caught in a high wind and fall to a lone shoulder-length strand that bears little relation to the rest of the hairstyle. Far better to accept that hair is not growing where it is wanted and cut and style the rest of the hair to make the best of this limitation.

Baldness in women

Women usually are not affected as badly as men, simply because their bodies do not produce the same level of androgen hormones. After the menopause there can be some loss of hair, usually seen between the ages of 55 and 60, but sometimes not until much later. Usually, the first signs are that the partings are thin; later, an oval-shaped bald patch can appear towards the back of the crown. Hormone replacement therapy may help, but it should be remembered that hormone treatment for hair loss is still in its infancy and a great deal of research still remains to be done by doctors and trichologists.

Baldness in children

Males under the age of puberty seldom go bald but, subsequently, the chances of this happening increase. Usually the hair loss develops symmetrically, starting at the temples and crown. It spreads gradually, while the circulating male hormones cause the scalp follicles to produce only short, very fine hairs.

Thinning hair sometimes affects teenagers, but when it does, it is rarely hormonal changes that are the cause. Stress is known to be a frequent cause of hair loss and is far more likely to be the underlying factor. The teenager may simply not be able to cope with the many pressures society imposes on our lives. One problem that can affect teenagers, and is more common with boys than girls, is excess secretion by the sebaceous glands, which can cause acné and a hair condition called *seborrhoea oleosa,* meaning oiliness of the scalp, often accompanied by hair loss.

Hairpieces and wigs

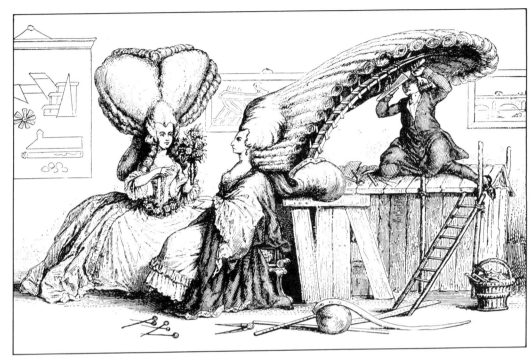

The height of fashion in wigs must surely have been reached just before the French Revolution. This humourous engraving of the day - 1788 - shows the hairdresser more in terms of a structural engineer than a hair stylist, building up a cantilevered superstructure with hammers, pliers and bricklayer's trowel, while the client gossips happily with a less 'well coiffured' companion.

The professional name given to a piece of false hair is 'postiche' and its function is by no means restricted to concealing thinning hair or baldness. In ancient Egypt and Rome, wigs were used on formal or festive occasions, worn by men and women over a clean-shaven scalp. Roman women liked to wear blond wigs, an obvious status symbol in a country where dark hair was the norm.

In the Middle Ages in Europe, wigs were frowned upon by the church – even when used for the purpose of hiding baldness. Any form of artificial adornment of the body was seen as wicked and regarded as a 'mark of the devil'. Not until the reign of Queen Elizabeth I did wig-wearing become accepted in England. The Queen had taken up wearing wigs when she lost her hair prematurely and is said to have owned some 80 wigs at the time of her death. Women's wigs in those days were often dyed red, in deference to Elizabeth who had red hair when she was young. Mary Queen of Scots had a collection of auburn wigs. When she was beheaded, it was quite a shock to those present to find out that the beautiful auburn tresses that she wore were not her own.

A hairpiece can take the form of a complete wig or a smaller hairpiece to cover only part of the scalp. Until the 1950s all hairpieces were made by hand, using a foundation, also known as a base, that was either soft and flexible or semi-rigid. When they became mass pro-ducted, stretch foundations were used, allowing the wearer simply to pull the wig over the scalp or hair.

A really good wig should look completely natural and fit snugly around the face and neck. With the finest quality wigs — those normally used to conceal baldness rather than for fashion purposes — it is not only the quality of the hair that matters, but the shape and fit of the foundation. To be really natural, a wig should not apply uneven pressure anywhere on the head. It should be both light and strong, so that it doesn't stretch quickly out of shape in wear.

Wigmaking is an art that involves not only the wigmaker, but also the hairdresser. This is because wigs should be cut and styled to suit your face, just as your own hair should be. This can be an exacting and lengthy business, so, to save time, the hairdresser sometimes first styles the wig on a malleable block, modelled on the shape of the back of the head.

To get that all-important secure fit, the wig specialist measures the client's head from several angles and then produces a template of the exact shape. Often several fittings are required to get the size absolutely right. It is not only the shape and size of the head that must be taken into account, but also the direction of the wearer's own hair growth. Once the wig or hairpiece is in place, it should be possible to comb out the hair in any direction without the foundation moving. When the hair is being used for wigmaking, it should also be attached to the foundation lying in the direction of the growth. This is because the overlapping scales of the hair shaft run smooth from root to point, but not vice versa.

How to choose a wig

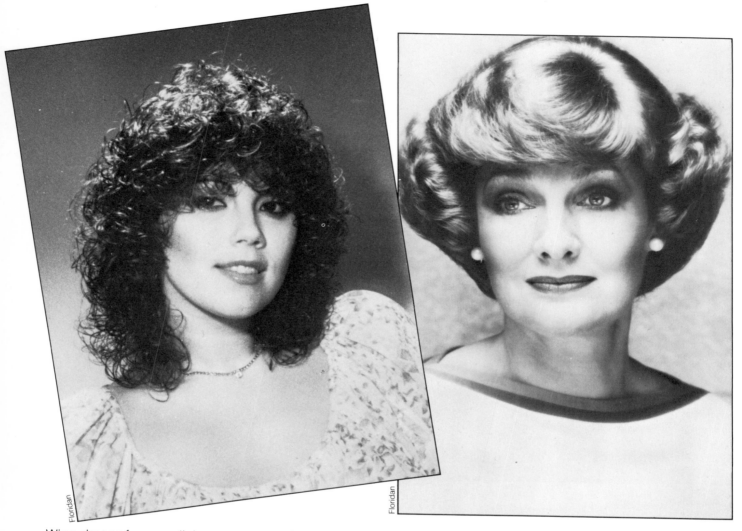

Floridan

Floridan

Wigs chosen for remedial purposes to replace a lost crop of hair and disguise a balding pate are generally hand-knotted and use hair that is a very close match to the wearer's own remaining hair. For this purpose, a hair sample for matching has to be taken from several areas on the head, that is, of course, if there's any hair left to be taken. Hair colour can vary even on one head and, by taking the different samples, the final hairpiece can be made to blend in closely with the surrounding hair.

Toupees for men are fastened to the scalp with double-sided adhesive tape. If the hairstyle demands a parting, the hair is knotted so as to lie either back or sideways from the parting. The knotting of the hair must look natural. Each hair must be well secured and often different varieties of hair are used – straight hair for the back and wavy or curly for the front. The result must also be in harmony with the crown hair which usually grows in a circular formation.

The knotted wig is the most natural and the most expensive to produce because it is entirely made by hand. Wigs in the medium price range are usually 'wefted'; this means they are machine made and are usually only finished by hand.

Most fibre wigs are pre-cut and ready to wear. Even so, a hairdresser can do a great deal to improve the look of a wig by trimming ragged ends or tapering the cut to suit the wearer's face. A wig can take years off you – and that is even if you have perfectly good natural hair! It can also be an enormous convenience, concealing less than perfect hair – or simply allowing you to pretend you're someone else for a little while. You don't even need to step out to the hairdressers to achieve a total transformation. There's only one snag: you really ought to take it off at night! If it is at all possible, occasionally give your head and scalp a break by leaving your wig off and spend a few days by yourself if necessary .

As you get older, shade mixing for a natural effect will become increasingly important. If hair loss has started,

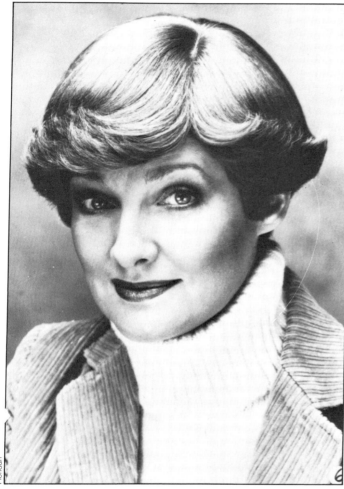

Floridan

The main advantage of a wig is its adaptability. By putting on a curly wig (far left) you can have a perm without the inconvenience of visiting your hairdresser. As Barbara Murray shows, a wig can completely alter your image - one minute you can look right for a candlelit dinner, and the next, sport a tomboy-look for the country with this flick-back style wig.

The two photographs below demonstrate the transformation that a toupee can make to a middle-aged man. This man has experienced almost complete hair loss at the crown of his head, which gives a straggly, unkempt look. The picture immediately below shows a radical improvement in the man's general appearance; he looks years younger and considerably more confident.

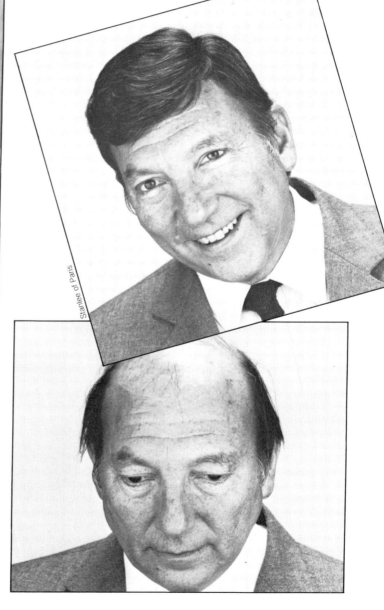

Stanlee of Paris

the hairdresser can make up a piece to fit in exactly with the area where thinning has occurred. Skilful fitting and trimming are essential so that the hairpiece is undetectible. Once in place, it can add extra height and fullness, giving a more youthful and fashionable appearance. Sometimes, especially when women lose some of their hair and the hairline is receding, a partial wig (wiglet) that covers only the front part of the scalp and tapers away to a point above or just behind the ears can be a good solution. Other times, a semi-wig (wiglet) will only cover the higher part of the forehead and top of the head.

Putting on a wig is extremely important and, here again, if you are uncertain, ask your hairdresser for advice. For a complete wig that totally covers the head, it is essential that the natural hair is first pinned away so that it doesn't slip out beneath the edge of the wig later. Always put the wig on front first, placing the centre of the front in the middle of the forehead and then holding it down while the wig is pulled on to the back of the neck.

The composition of wigs

Wigs are made of any of three different types of material: European hair, Asian hair or synthetic fibre. For wigs that are worn daily, nothing beats the quality and appearance of real hair. European hair is generally considered to be the very finest available, having a much better texture than Asian hair and very much better texture than synthetic fibre. Another advantage of European hair is that it is available in a wide range of natural shades, from light blond to black. Therefore, a wig or hairpiece made of European hair can usually be kept in its own natural colour, rather than be dyed or bleached.

Natural hair

Hair collecting used to be rather a haphazard business and hair pedlars were a common sight in Europe, where peasants could part with their locks for an agreed sum of money. To this day in Italy, brides are known to raise money for their dowry by selling their hair. The most valuable of all natural hair shades is pure white, followed by blond and reddish hair. Blond hair is often collected in Germany and the Scandinavian countries, whereas the best quality dark hair is supposed to come from Spain and Italy. France is credited with producing the best brown and auburn hair.

To obtain a natural-looking match, it is often necessary to mix different shades. If the exact shade is unavailable, the wigmaker can use hair that is a tone lighter and mix it with a tone that is darker. Grey or white hair may have to be added if the client's hair is greying. In brown hair, there are frequently red or yellow and sometimes even ashy tones that need to be blended with the predominant shade.

Asian hair in its natural state only comes in two shades, black or brown. Therefore, if you buy an Asian hair wig, and it comes in any other colour, you can be sure that it will have been treated with some drastic dyeing process. A vast proportion of wigs are imported ready-made from the Far East. Asian hair is much coarser than European hair, so the texture is often refined with chemical processes. With all the treatments the hair has undergone, it is usually not a good idea to subject an Asian wig to further hairdressing processes.

Synthetic fibres

Great strides have been made in synthetic fibres, but it must be admitted that nothing as yet looks and handles exactly as real human hair. Although the external appearance may be similar, the structure, for example, of an acrylic fibre differs totally from natural hair. For one thing, it does not have the cuticle scales layer. And it is important to note here that tinting, bleaching or perming should never be done on synthetic fibre hair.

The first synthetic fibre used for wigs was made of nylon, nylon blends or acetates. In looks and texture, it left a great deal to be desired: often it was unnaturally shiny, with a coarse but fly-away texture. It was difficult to keep clean as washing would often result in tangling.

The acrylics used subsequently were an enormous improvement, and looked very natural. These wigs were easy to wash and the style would bounce back naturally after drying. What is more, these wigs were relatively inexpensive, being very much cheaper than Asian hair. In the early 1970s, synthetic fibre hair had improved to such an extent that it had even adopted a natural hair's cuticle-type surface.

There are many quality variations in fibre wigs and often the snags are not immediately apparent. Some wigs look nice, but can feel rather coarse and unpleasant. If this is the case, think twice before buying. If the hair texture feels wrong, the wig may not hold its style for any length of time. A good wig must be well shaped. Avoid those that look bulky with hair standing away at the nape. A good fibre looks beautiful in any light. Inferior wigs often look pleasant in daylight, but have a glittery unnatural appearance the minute you are in bright, artificial light. Take a close look at the way the hair is joined at the base. Unless the gaps are narrow and the hair is full, the base can show through the strands.

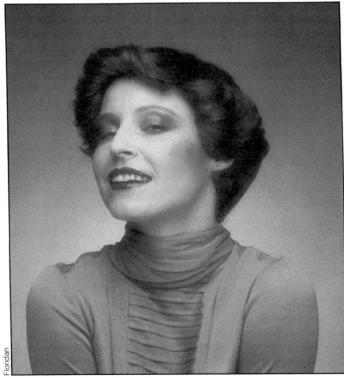

Above: *Make sure that your wig looks and feels as natural as possible.*

146

Washing and care of wigs

Unless you have a synthetic fibre wig that is clearly labelled as 'washable' when you buy it, it is usually best to have wigs and hairpieces made out of human hair cleaned professionally. This is because, unless the hairs are really firmly anchored in the base, water can loosen them. Even in the dry-cleaning process, care must be taken over the method used. Cleaning should not adversely affect the base or foundation of the wig, which needs to be very carefully protected from distortion or other damage.

The first step, therefore, is to mount the wig or hairpiece on an appropriate malleable block before brushing a special wig-cleaning fluid through the hair with a soft brush. Alternatively, the hairpiece can be sprayed with cleaning fluid and brushed out over a bowl afterwards. The dry-cleaning fluid contains a grease solvent that will normally remove dirt and grease, but sometimes, if a wig has been left to get very dirty, the whole hairpiece may have to be immersed in the cleaning fluid. This is, of course, the last resort, as you should really try to avoid getting any of the cleaning fluid on to the foundation.

A word of warning. Always take care when using any kind of wig cleaning fluid because the fumes are toxic and should not be inhaled. So, when cleaning your wig or hairpiece, never use the fluid when in a confined space where the fumes can build up; always clean your wig in a well ventilated room.

If you really care about the condition of your wig, you are well advised to have it cleaned often. A soiled wig, like dirty hair, will become limp and lustreless and, the longer you leave it, the harder it will be to restore to its former gloss. Even when you hand-wash a synthetic fibre wig, you should take care not to wet the foundation more than you need to. A bowl of warm water to which you have added a little mild shampoo is all you need. Simply dip the hair into the bowl, working in the lather gently, having first combed out the wig to ensure there are no tangles.

Never actually rub the hair, as this can cause tangles or knots. When you have washed the wig, several times if necessary, rinse well in clean warm water. If you are using a hand shower, let the water trickle down from root to point.

Sometimes, professional wig cleaners will use the washing method for real hair wigs and hairpieces, especially when these have a stretch foundation. The hairpiece is rinsed after washing in water with a little conditioner added, before being rinsed in clear water. Sometimes the hairpiece is then left to dry naturally and re-dampened for setting.

The advantage of wigs or hairpieces made of European hair is that the hairdresser can work on them in just the same way as on living hair. If the hair needs to be re-coloured, it is normal for a colour test to be done first. On the whole, a drastic colour change is not recom-mended and the dye must not be allowed to come in contact with the foundation, as it can cause it to rot. As some hairpieces contain both natural and fake hair, careful checking has to be carried out to avoid any damaging effects. The wig should never be removed from the malleable block until it is completely dry, to prevent the base from shrinking.

Perming wigs

A perm can change a straight-hair wig into a fashionable curly style, but, once again, the type of wig will determine just how much treatment it can stand. Because it has probably been pre-bleached, the Asian wig can usually only stand a cold perm that has been specially formulated for bleached hair. Colouring is usually a safer process because the chemicals are milder than permanent wave lotions, and a wig that looks a little 'tired' or faded can benefit from a tint or rinse to perk it up.

As wig hair doesn't grow, it should be remembered that mistakes are costly: once the wig has been wrongly cut, coloured or permed, it is usually impossible to correct the error afterwards.

If you buy a wig off-the-rack, always check carefully what you can or cannot do with it. Some acrylic types are so easy that you can literally put them in the washing machine and hang them up to dry. Others react badly to heat and will melt if you try to set them with heated rollers. Acrylic wigs may not look that natural, but they can be fun fashion accessories. However, never forget that your own hair has to live underneath and it is not a good idea to have it covered for days on end.

Useful advice

With wigs, there are some disadvantages to be consi-dered and before you decide to start wearing a hairpiece, you should take note of the following points. Once people have become used to your wig, and this is particularly so with balding men, they will gradually come to accept the hairpiece as part of your natural appearance. This means that you will find it very difficult to wear it one day and leave it off the next. Wearing a wig will mean continuous expense: for men wearing a toupee, for example, it not only means a regular cleaning fee, but the cost of sticky tape essential for keeping the wig in place. Wigs can fade or discolour in sunlight, and they can be very hot. They can also come loose if perspiration of the scalp dislodges the tape.

Most important of all, take care to choose a wig to suit you and your personality. If you have had thinning, sparse hair for years, your friends will find it odd – to say the least – when you suddenly turn up with a thick and bushy crown.

Transplants

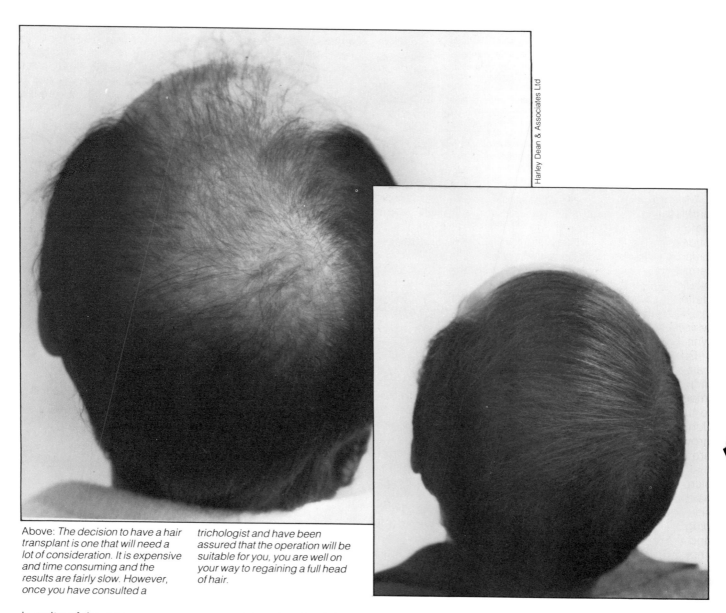

Harley Dean & Associates Ltd

Above: *The decision to have a hair transplant is one that will need a lot of consideration. It is expensive and time consuming and the results are fairly slow. However, once you have consulted a* *trichologist and have been assured that the operation will be suitable for you, you are well on your way to regaining a full head of hair.*

In spite of the enormous expense and time involved, hair transplants are becoming more popular. The idea of wearing someone else's hair, rather than your own, is not very attractive to many people – even if this hair looks natural enough. There is always the fear that a sudden gust of wind will dislodge the wig or toupee, and there are also those inconvenient restrictions such as not allowing the hair to get wet. Hair transplant operations can solve all these problems – at a price.

If you are considering having a hair transplant, it is really necessary to consult a recognized trichologist for advice first. Also remember that surgical hair replacement operations are making small fortunes for some

unscrupulous operators, so make sure that you have some sound unbiased facts at your fingertips. Remember also that, because you are undergoing a surgical procedure, a full medical check-up should precede it, including a blood test. Make sure the clinic or hospital where you are staying is registered, and that you know exactly what to expect and to do after the operation. Many clinics or hospitals adopt a rather casual approach to transplants, because it is thought that, as the operation is not a major one, patients will not be in any need of advice. Of course, this is not true. By all means demand attention, if necessary.

Ask the trichologist if there is an alternative to hair

transplantation, which is still a fairly drastic treatment. Some dietary advice may not come amiss at this stage and a course of scalp massage treatments could help loosen a tight scalp, stimulate the blood flow and have a stimulating effect on the hair follicles. Many men have found that massage, combined with scrupulous hair care and hygiene, can slow down hair loss and even prevent it to some extent. But this is usually just practising delaying tactics, welcome as they are. Eventually the amount of hair will lessen and the pattern of baldness will become evident.

Medical research is involved with the development of anti-androgen pills to block the action of the male hormones which cause hair loss, but so far the adverse effects are unacceptable: apart from headaches, blushing and sweating, men have put on weight, with a female distribution of fat. Given the choice, most men would agree that, in the circumstances, hair loss is definitely the lesser evil.

There are basically two techniques: the original method which is known as punch grafting and the latest technique which is called the flap-rotation method.

Basically, with punch grafting, small cylinders of hair-bearing skin are taken from a donor site and placed in 'punched-out' sites situated in a bald area. As you can imagine, both the donor site and the recipient areas have to be marked out carefully. What is more, the hair on the donor site is cut short first, so that the angle of the hair growth can be established. Then, after the hair and scalp are thoroughly washed, a local anaesthetic is injected to make the area numb. The punch is used to penetrate the skin on the scalp at the right angle, so as to catch as many hairs as possible in each graft. Then a plug consisting of skin and hair, (the donor plug) is removed and a recipient plug is cut. The donor plug is placed in the recipient site and must be level with the surrounding skin. It is also important to make sure that the hair faces in the right direction to blend with the hairstyle. After this, the head is bandaged.

After a few hours' rest, the patient can usually leave the surgery and is given a supply of antibiotics to prevent infection. After-care is important.

The scalp must be kept clean and water should be allowed to run over the punch grafts the day following the operation. After a few days, the hair can be shampooed as usual. Around 50 plugs are transferred in one sitting. Usually, the only ill effects are a headache for a day or so. Within one week, small crusts normally form around the graft and, after about three weeks, the transplanted hairs are shed, but re-grow a month or two later. The sections of implanted hair will continue to produce hair that grows to a normal length, with the same colour, texture and strength as it did in the original donor area.

At further sessions, the areas between the grafts are fitted in until all the bald areas have been replaced by hair-bearing grafts. After a few months, the donor sites should have completely healed, and only very slight scars will still be visible. Because the punches from the donor site will have been taken from areas of the head where the hair is growing thickly – usually at the back of the head and nape of the neck – and taken in widely-spaced punches, the loss of hair in this area will not be noticeable and the minute bald patches will be easily covered by the remaining natural growth. The best news of all is that, performed by a qualified surgeon, the success rate is around 95 per cent.

The flap-rotation method

The flap-rotation technique is also performed under a local anaesthetic and is usually done in two stages, with a delay of seven days between each stage. With this technique, a flap of up to 2½ inches (6.3 centimetres) wide and around 8 inches (20 centimetres) long from a hair-growing area is transplanted to a bald patch. Each flap contains between 8 and 10,000 hairs, in contrast to the average single punch graft yielding 8 to 15 hairs. As the base of the flap – which has a tongue-like shape – is not severed, the flap of hair-producing skin continues to have its own blood supply and therefore survives until the graft has taken.

In punch grafting, there is a three-month delay before the regrowth shows. With the flap-rotation technique, the hair does not fall out and it continues growing throughout the procedure so a good head of hair is immediately apparent.

However, not many heads of hair can take the flap rotation technique. The flap has to be cut from a section where hair is plentiful, and where there is sufficient growth for the patch that has been taken away to be covered by hair growing over the area. A certain shrinkage of the zone where the flap has been cut as it heals over will reduce the amount of disguise necessary, but nonetheless the possibilities of the operation have to be skilfully assessed to ensure that there is no obvious bald patch left at the donor site.

Scalp reduction

There is a third option, not actually hair transplantation, which can help reduce bald patches known as scalp reduction. An incision is made down the centre of the bald patch and the skin and fatty tissues are trimmed away. Then the scalp is sewn up, reducing the bald patch. As the skin on the scalp is elastic, a number of these operations can be done over a period of time, until the bald patch disappears. Sometimes scalp reduction is combined with punch grafting to give an overall covering.

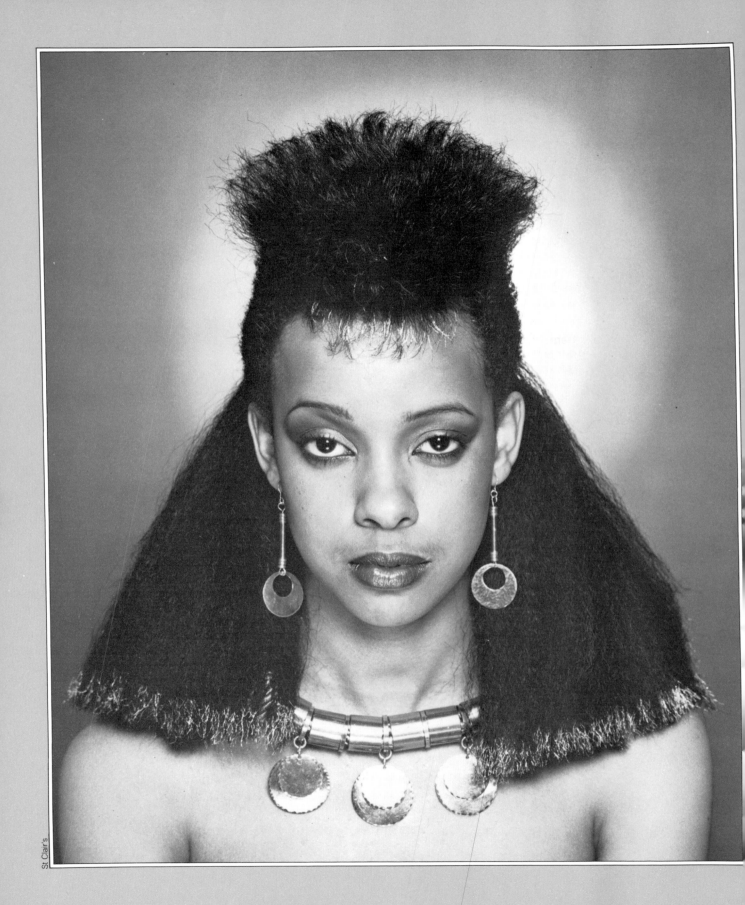

Conclusion

In this book, many facets of hair have been looked at in detail: what it is, keeping it healthy, washing, drying, styling, cutting, colouring, waving it, straightening it, dressing it up, thinning hair, hair problems and even recipes for do-it-yourself shampoos and conditioners.

The title of this book – *Hair Magic* – was deliberate. It was *Hair Magic* because magic implies seemingly supernatural transformations; dramatic changes happening at the wave of a wand with you or your hairdresser as the magician.

Healthy hair and a healthy scalp, along with a good haircut, are the basic magic ingredients of any hairstyle. All other elements, such as perms, colours, tipping and accessories, can be added later on to make sure that the overall effect is one that agrees with your lifestyle and the particular occasion.

Hair Magic has, it is hoped, shown what you can achieve with your hair and what your hairdresser, with your help, can achieve with it. Hairdressing is a skilled and complex art. Good hairdressers are skilled and professional artists and it is very unlikely that you will be able to reproduce their achievements – especially on your own head of hair – if what you require is an intricate style. Remember, you can never actually see your hair. If you are styling your own it all has to be done with mirrors and this in itself requires a number of skills that are not necessarily easy to learn.

A good hairdresser need not be the most fashionable or the most expensive but one who has an empathy with you, is on your wavelength, and is able to understand what *you* are trying to achieve with your hair even though you yourself cannot express exactly what you want in words, or might not even be consciously aware of what you are looking for.

Do not be intimidated by your hairdresser. Some years ago it seemed that the more expensive and fashionable salons treated their clients – with a few favoured exceptions – with a disregard that almost bordered on the discourteous. They were dictatorial in their choice of style and kept clients waiting for unnecessary lengths of time. Fortunately, that way of operating now seems to be fast disappearing, probably because dissatisfied customers sensibly voted with their feet and left. Such salons were left to face the harsh winds of economic reality – which require that the needs of the customer come first.

A visit to the hairdresser should be something to look forward to, a pleasurable experience from which you will emerge looking and, consequently, feeling better. If you regard the experience as less than pleasurable, then change your hairdresser. You, after all, are doing the salon a favour by giving your custom and your money.

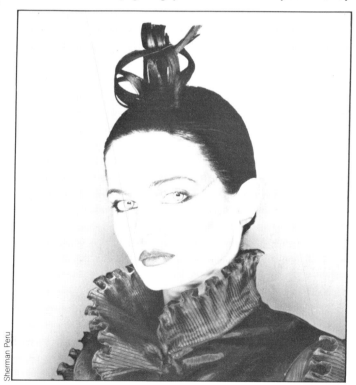

Sherman Peru

Left: *The sides are cut close, leaving the hair at the nape long. Glitter is brushed on to the tips of the hair.*

Above: *Plenty of gel has been used to create this elaborate hairstyle. The result is a dramatic, but glamorous evening look.*

The salon is not paying you.

As you will have noticed, this is not a book for the do-it-yourself hairdresser, even though there are many do-it-yourself ideas contained within its pages. It is a book intended to help you work *with* your hairdresser to find the magic which resides in your hair and to use it to promote the full potential of your total look.

Work *with* your hair; don't fight it. You cannot make your hair in to what it is not, but you can work wonders with it if you appreciate its limitations. You must try to get the best out of what you do have rather than wishing in vain for something you will never have.

Be practical. Remember that your hair needs to fit in with your lifestyle. If you have plenty of time and money to spend on yourself and your hair, you can go to your hairdressers frequently and can perhaps afford elaborate hairstyles. However, if you've got a full-time job, four kids, no money and a broken down car then you almost undoubtedly need to keep it as simple as possible. Hairstyles in fashion magazines are, as often as not, for fantasy people rather than for others like ourselves. These fantasy people maintain themselves with the aid of lacquers, off-camera pins, grips and other hairdressing hardware, two photographers' assistants and a make-up artist for as long as it takes to shoot a photograph. After they have finished their photograph session, as likely as not they will let their hair down, put their feet up and have a cup of tea!

Most leading manufacturers of hair products have departments which are available to provide advice and assistance to the general public to get the best results from the products they use. Don't hesitate to make use of these facilities, and remember that this advice, which comes free of charge, is one of the advantages of using well-known brands rather than cheaper substitutes.

Unlike a lot of beauty preparations, with hair care products you tend to get what you pay for. When buying hair products it is sensible to buy your purchases at your salon, which will usually have on sale a range of products that are used and recommended and will be particularly suited to your specific needs. The one disadvantage of buying hair care preparations from your hairdresser is that they will very probably be more expensive than similar preparations at chemists or department stores.

Nevertheless, even if you don't buy your hair care products from your hairdresser, ask for, and take, professional advice. Hairdressers are experts who, generally speaking, will have no particular product axe to grind. They can direct you to suitable product types rather than to specific brand names.

Almost all hair products can be used to great advantage by men as well as women. Admittedly, some of the fragrances embedded in hair care products appear to have a rather overpowering odour and to be aimed at women rather than men. But today there is a general awareness of the importance of hair care for men, which for a long time has been very neglected. There are many hair care products aimed specifically at men – and very many which have no smell at all. So don't be frightened into using a product which might make you smell of a French beauty salon... you don't have to buy such products.

The widespread availability of a very wide range of both temporary and permanent hair colourants has revolutionized hair fashion. Bizarre punk hairstyles may not be to your taste but, without question, they have impact. Done well, they can be superb to look at and at their best are almost an art form. They are the ultimate expression of the amateur hairdresser. You may not wish to emulate the extremes of punk high fashion but more and more elements of these street styles are being adapted and used by the hairdressing establishments for an up-to-date and discerning clientele. You can be bold, use colours or spray-on designs (there are some superb ideas and templates on pages 160 and 161). Try out your own ideas with ragbands, butterfly clips, chopsticks, combs, ribbons, jewelry, soft belts, tiaras or even coat-hangers. The list is endless, limited only by your imagination.

Hair care and hair styling are, or should be, especially important to those who are going bald. In this era of the cult of youth the stress caused by any incipient sign of baldness is often enough to make one's hair fall out through worrying about it. For those who are bald at the moment, or may be going bald, don't despair. Bald is, or can be, beautiful.

Nowadays there is more concern than ever before for our hair and hair care. But, and this has been said many time throughout the book, you cannot have healthy hair without being healthy, and if your hair looks good and feels good then *you* will look good and feel good. Therefore, two things are essential. The first is that you should lead a healthy life, with plenty of exercise and a good diet – and this means going without cigarettes and not drinking an excessive amount of alcohol. This way you will almost undoubtedly achieve a healthy growth of hair. The second point to note is that you must somehow find the time to care for your hair properly, either by going to a hairdresser or by taking care of your hair yourself. It is no good if you are healthy as can be and don't bother with your hair. You will look as bad as someone who smokes 100 cigarettes, and drinks a bottle of whisky, a day.

We hope you have enjoyed this book. You may have read it right through very carefully or may have just dipped into it to get some ideas and inspirations. Above all, we hope we have helped you to get enjoyment and fun from your hair and that you have found the secret of Hair Magic.

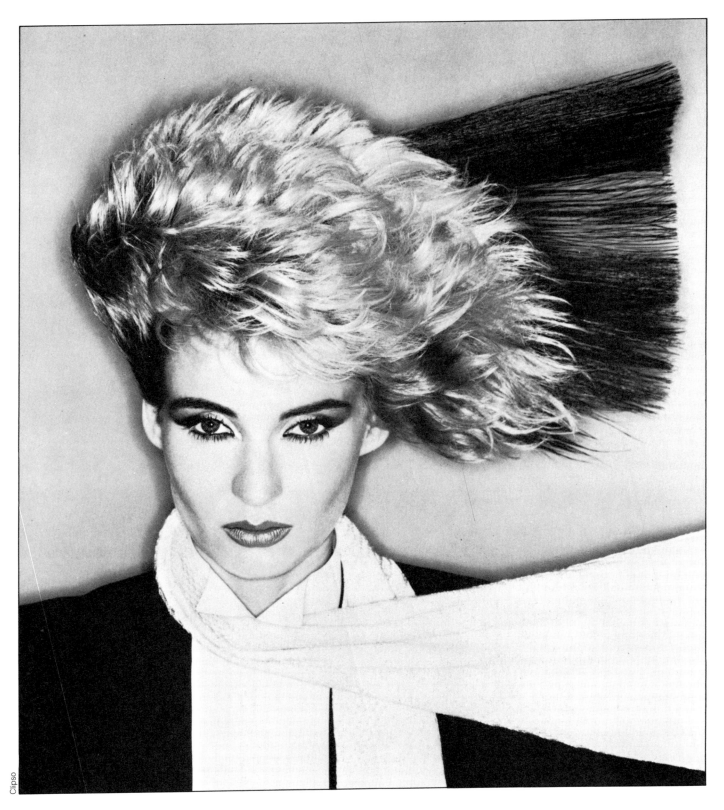

Clipso

153

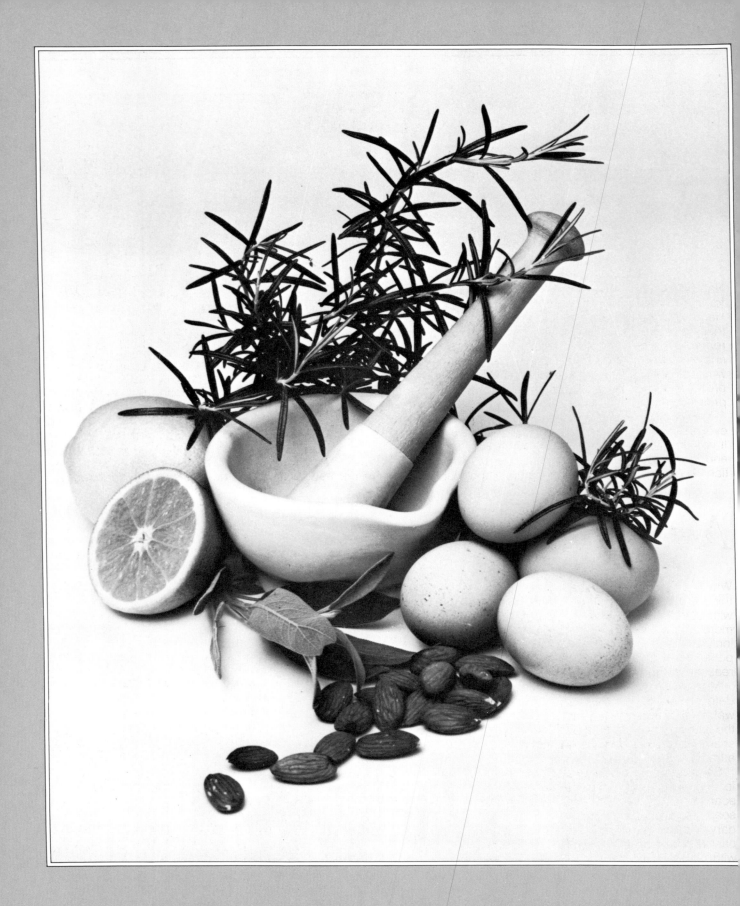

Recipes

Natural products have been used for thousands of years for their healing, soothing and beautifying properties. Herbs, flowers and oils have established a reputation for their curative and beautifying qualities. Until quite recently, mother nature was relied upon to provide all hair and skin care treatments so there should be little wonder why so many people are turning either to commercial products which have a large proportion of natural products, or, indeed, to home made beauty care aids.

Many hair care preparations are very easy to make and even the most complicated take only little time to prepare. If you decide to invest a little effort you can save money and obtain the satisfaction of making your own preparation, knowing that only pure, natural ingredients have been used. In addition, once you become familiar with the ingredients and formulations, you can gradually adjust the preparation to suit your own needs.

There are only a few simple precautions to take as none of the ingredients of any of the preparations are dangerous. If the instructions require the use of heat, make sure you take the normal safety precautions, especially if you are adding natural oils to a mixture. It is also wise to test each formulation on a piece of out-of-the-way sample hair, in case it is not quite right for you. Remember, your hair condition changes with your physical and emotional health, and that this may effect the result you get from any hair preparation; however, with milder natural products the risk is usually reduced.

Natural Shampoos

When concocting shampoos yourself at home, the first thing to bear in mind is that you are not trying to compete with commercial brands, some of which contain 100 or more ingredients. Your home-made variety will not include the preservatives present in shop-bought shampoos, so whatever you make should be used up reasonably quickly, preferably within a few days.

Modern commercial shampoos are mostly made with detergents rather than with soaps. The major ingredient is water which is combined with a foaming agent to improve the lather, and often a perfume is added. Ideally, a shampoo should leave the hair not only clean but with an attractive shine, fragrance and texture.

Soap can be a useful base in home-made shampoos for loosening dirt and degreasing the hair, but not all soaps are suitable for this purpose. As making your own soap involves the use of caustic soda, which is dangerous to handle, the best thing is to buy a few bars of castile soap or castile soap flakes. Castile soap is made with olive oil and soda. It has a hard, close grain and contains only a little water. The bars should be grated prior to use.

Herb Shampoo

For 4-6 shampoo applications

1oz (25g) fresh camomile, rosemary or sage
20 fl oz (600 ml) water
1oz (25g) grated castile soap

Infuse the herbs in cold water overnight. Strain them through muslin and heat the water the herbs have been infused in in an enamel saucepan, together with the grated soap. Heat and stir, until the soap has melted. Remove from heat and allow to cool. If the soap solidifies, put the container in a warm place until it re-melts and then give it a good shake.

If dried herbs are used, reduce the quantity used by half. The ingredients should mean that the mixture will keep fresh for a few weeks.

Different herbs suit different types of hair. So be careful to select the herb that is best for you. Below is a table which lists types of hair and the particular herbs required.

TYPE OF HAIR	HERB
Dry	Sage or elderflower
Oily	Mint, lavender or marigold
Scurfy or Dandruffy	Rosemary

Egg Shampoo

For 1 shampoo application

1 or 2 eggs
8 fl oz (225ml) warm water

Beat 1 or 2 eggs in the warm water and massage into the wet hair. Leave on the hair for about 10 minutes and then rinse thoroughly with water.

This recipe is for all hair types.

Egg Shampoo with Bay Rum and Rose-water Rinse

For 1 shampoo application

4 eggs
8 fl oz (225ml) rose-water
8 fl oz (225ml) bay rum

Beat the eggs and massage them into the wet hair. Leave for 15 minutes and then rinse thoroughly with water.

Mix the rose-water and rum and pour over the hair to give a thorough rinse.

This recipe is for oily hair.

Egg Yolk Shampoo

For 1 shampoo application

2 egg yolks
8 fl oz (225ml) warm water

Beat the egg yolks in warm water and massage into the wet hair for 5 minutes. Then leave for a further 10 minutes. Rinse thoroughly with water.

This shampoo may leave the hair with a slightly unpleasant smell. A final rinse, using orange-water, rose-water or an infusion of rose petal, is advisable.

For all hair types.

Egg and Herb Shampoo

For 1 shampoo application

1 egg
½oz (15g) herbs
8 fl oz (225ml) boiling water

Infuse the herbs in boiling water. When cool, strain through muslin. Use camomile if you have light coloured hair, or rosemary or sage if it is dark.

Separate the egg and beat the yolk for dry hair, or the white of egg if you have oily hair, into the infusion.

Massage into wet hair and rinse with water.

Egg and Orange Shampoo

For 2 shampoo applications

1 egg yolk
1 tablespoon (15ml) orange juice
½oz (15g) soapwort root
20 fl oz (600ml) boiling water

Infuse the soapwort root in boiling water and then leave for 15 minutes. Strain through muslin and add the egg yolk and orange juice to the infusion and beat to a smooth consistency.

Massage into wet hair, leave for 10 minutes and then rinse with water.

For all hair types.

Anti-Dandruff Shampoo

For 1 shampoo application

2 egg yolks
12 fl oz (340ml) warm water
2 teaspoons (10ml) vinegar

In order to give this shampoo a pleasanter smell add 1 drop of lavender oil or concentrated perfume to the mixture.

Beat the egg yolks into 4 fl oz (115ml) warm water. Massage the mixture well into the scalp and then leave for about 10 minutes. Rinse with warm water.

Add vinegar to 8 fl oz (225ml) of cool, rather than cold, water and use as a rinse. Rinse the hair two or three times.

Camomile Shampoo

For 2-3 shampoo applications

2oz (50g) fresh camomile
20 fl oz (600ml) boiling water
2 teaspoons (10ml) lemon juice
4oz (100g) grated castile soap

Infuse the camomile in boiling water. Allow to cool and then add the lemon juice. Add grated soap and bring to the boil, stirring all the time.

This shampoo is for blond hair.

Conditioners

To keep your hair looking sleek and smooth and to keep it feeling soft, it is necessary to use regular conditioning treatments. The best way of replacing the moisture that has been lost as a result of the harsh environmental factors of everyday life is to apply natural conditioners, such as warm oil and protein packs, to your hair.

Oil Conditioner

Warm oil makes an excellent conditioner for both hair and scalp. You can use any vegetable oil you have available; some, however, are particularly suitable. Olive oil is good for dry, brittle hair and castor oil has a beneficial effect on hair that is fragile and split. Almond oil and lavender oil are beneficial for all hair types and jo-joba oil can be used to treat damaged, curly and coarse hair.

Simply warm a little oil, then part the hair into sections and massage it into hair and scalp, combing through to ensure it penetrates thoroughly.

Immerse a clean towel in water, which is as hot as you can comfortably handle, then wring it to squeeze out as much of the water as possible. Wrap the head in the steaming towel to drive the oil into the hair and scalp. Keep the towel as steamy as possible by regularly re-immersing it in hot water and wringing it out. Preferably use two towels so the head can be 'steamed', using each towel alternately. Continue this process for 30 minutes. Alternatively, wrap your hair in clingfilm and soak in a hot, steamy bath.

Oil is used as the basis of many natural conditioners. The addition of eggs and honey, in particular, make an even more effective conditioner.

Honey and Olive Oil Conditioner

For 2 applications

8 fl oz (225ml) liquid honey
4 fl oz (115ml) olive oil

Put both of the ingredients into a screw-top container and shake thoroughly. Allow to blend for a day, periodically shaking the container.

When ready, massage into hair and scalp and cover with a plastic bag or clingfilm and leave for 30 minutes. Then shampoo.

This conditioner is suitable for dark hair.

Egg, Honey and Sesame Oil Conditioner

For 1 application

1 egg
1 teaspoon (5ml) honey
2 teaspoons (10ml) sesame oil

Add the honey to the oil, which has been gently heated in a saucepan with a water jacket (bain-marie). Beat the egg and add it slowly to the honey and oil mixture, stirring continuously.

Massage well into the hair and leave for 30 minutes. Cover the hair with a plastic bag to retain the heat. Then shampoo.

This conditioner is suitable for all hair types.

Egg and Coconut Oil Conditioner

For 1 application

1 egg
2 tablespoons (30ml) coconut oil
1 tablespoon (15ml) vinegar

The coconut oil should be heated gently before adding the beaten egg and vinegar. Use the preparation while it is warm to ensure that it stays a liquid. Massage into your hair. Keep your head covered for 30 minutes with a steaming towel, as described above, to ensure proper penetration of the conditioner. Then shampoo.

This conditioner is suitable for all hair types.

Protein conditioner with eggs

For 1 application

2 eggs
1 tablespoon (15ml) olive oil
1 tablespoon (15ml) glycerine
1 teaspoon (5ml) vinegar

Beat the eggs, and add the olive oil and glycerine slowly, while mixing. Add the vinegar. Wash hair once with shampoo, rinse, then massage in the conditioner. Leave for 30 minutes covering the hair with a plastic bag. Then shampoo hair again.

This conditioner is suitable for all hair types.

Last minute conditioners

Rosemary and Macassar oil may be used as last minute conditioners before you complete your hair preparations. Add a few drops of rosemary oil to your brush before brushing your hair. If you are using Macassar oil as a conditioner rub a few drops into your hair with your hands. Be careful with Macassar oil — it has notorious staining properties.

If you have any home-made mayonnaise left over it will make an excellent conditioner since it combines those marvellous ingredients eggs and oil. Also an avocado, when liquidized, can be used as a conditioner.

Rinses

Rinsing preparations are meant to be used as a final rinse after a shampoo and a water rinse. They give your hair a pleasing fragrance, enhance hair colour and encourage shine. Choose the rinse that suits your hair colour and condition.

Darkening rinse

For 1 application

2oz (50g) sage leaves
20 fl oz (600ml) boiling water

Sage has long been popular for brunettes to add shine and give back depth of colour to dark hair that has a faded look. It also has a mildly acidic content that helps keep the hair in good condition. Add a generous handful of sage leaves to the boiling water, allow the water to cool and then strain off the liquid through fine butter muslin or a coffee filter paper. Catch the liquid in a bowl and re-strain several times. Leave the sage water on the hair until it is almost dry before setting or drying the hair. Rosemary will substitute for sage.

This conditioner is suitable for brunette hair.

Lightening rinse

For 1 application

2oz (50g) camomile flowers
20 fl oz (600ml) boiling water

Camomile is well known as a hair lightener, suiting light brown to fair hair which is dry to normal. Infuse the camomile flowers for about 30 minutes in the boiling water. Allow the infusion to cool and strain off, as for a darkening rinse (above). Broom flowers and petals make a good substitute for camomile. Add a little quince juice for shine.

This conditioner is suitable for blond hair.

Nettle rinse

For 1 application

6 nettle stalks
40 fl oz (1.1 litres) boiling water
1 tablespoon (15ml) lemon juice or vinegar

The common nettle (*Urtica Urens*) can be used to make a general purpose rinse to promote hair health, and is said to be particularly beneficial if you are trying to eliminate dandruff or dry hair.

Pick 6 large nettle stalks; rinse thoroughly under cold water to remove dust and earth and then pick off the leaves. Infuse the leaves in the boiling water until the water is warm. Strain and use as final rinse. Place a bowl under your hair and re-use.

You can add vinegar or lemon juice to a rinse to help restore the acid mantle of the hair. Vinegar is best for dark hair and lemon for fair. If you want to lighten your hair you should sit in the sun after using the rinse. The vinegar smell soon disappears so don't worry. Add 1 tablespoon (15ml) of whichever suits your hair to about 8 times the amount of rinse solution.

A cold rinse will help the pores of the scalp close and make the hair shiny.

Reddening rinse

For 1 application

1 tablespoon (15ml) henna
10 fl oz (300ml) warm water

Henna can be used to prepare a rinse as well as a full strength colourant. Add the henna powder to the warm water.

Marigold and privet give coppery highlights in brown, red and fair hair. As for other herbs, infuse a handful in 20 fl oz (600ml) of boiling water, allow to cool and strain off the plant material.

Colourants

The best known and most powerful colourant is henna. A reddish-brown powder is obtained from the leaf of an oriental shrub. The best henna is imported from Egypt. Its colouring effect varies according to strength, treatment time and the natural colour of your hair. It is safe because it is non toxic, but its strength means you must experiment before you use it. Compared with henna, other colourants are much weaker and require several applications.

Basic Henna

For 1 application

8oz (225g) henna
1 teaspoon (5ml) vinegar
8 fl oz (225ml) water

Warm the water and add the henna powder slowly while mixing to make a thick paste. Add the vinegar and allow to stand for 1 hour. Re-warm in a saucepan with a water jacket and apply with gloved hands to the hair, which has already been sectioned. After combing the paste through, cover your hair in a plastic bag and leave for 30 minutes. Check the hair colour and leave for further periods of 30 minutes until the desired colour is achieved. The longer the hair is left the stronger the colour will be. For a really strong colour leave the henna on all night, if possible. When you are satisfied with the colour, wash your hair and rinse until the water is clear.

To redden hair.

Henna and Tea

For 1 application

8oz (225g) henna
1 tablespoon (15ml) Indian tea or red sage
24 fl oz (775ml) boiling water

Infuse the tea in 16 fl oz (450ml) of boiling water for 2 hours. When cool, filter off the leaves and add the liquid slowly to the henna to make a paste. If necessary add part or all of a further cup of warm water to make the paste malleable.

Apply to sections of the hair with gloved hands, cover, check and wash, as above.

The tea (or red sage) subdues the red tones to give an auburn effect.

For a subdued red tone.

Henna and Camomile

For 1 application

8oz (225g) henna
8oz (225g) camomile flowers
24 fl oz (775ml) boiling water
1 teaspoon (5ml) vinegar

Infuse the camomile in boiling water for at least two hours, then add the vinegar. Filter away any vegetable matter from the infusion and add slowly to the henna powder to form a malleable paste, as described above. The camomile lightens the reddening effect.

To restore colour to fading brown hair.

Camomile

As camomile is very much weaker than henna it is necessary to make several applications to obtain any lightening effect. First make a strong infusion of camomile, as described above, and make this into a malleable paste, using kaolin powder. The kaolin simply makes the paste and has no colouring effect. Apply to the hair as for henna and leave for 1 hour with the hair covered with a plastic bag.

Rinse with warm water. Repeat to achieve the desired degree of lightening.

Setting lotions

There are several old-fashioned 'kitchen cupboard' aids for setting hair. Beer, light ale preferably, should be used when it is 'flat' so the chemicals in it will have dissipated; fresh milk is good for anyone with dry hair, whilst powdered skimmed milk made up with water is best for greasy hair and neat lemon juice is also good for greasy, as well as fair, hair. Simply apply to freshly shampooed hair that has been towel dried and set in the usual way.

Colour magic stencils

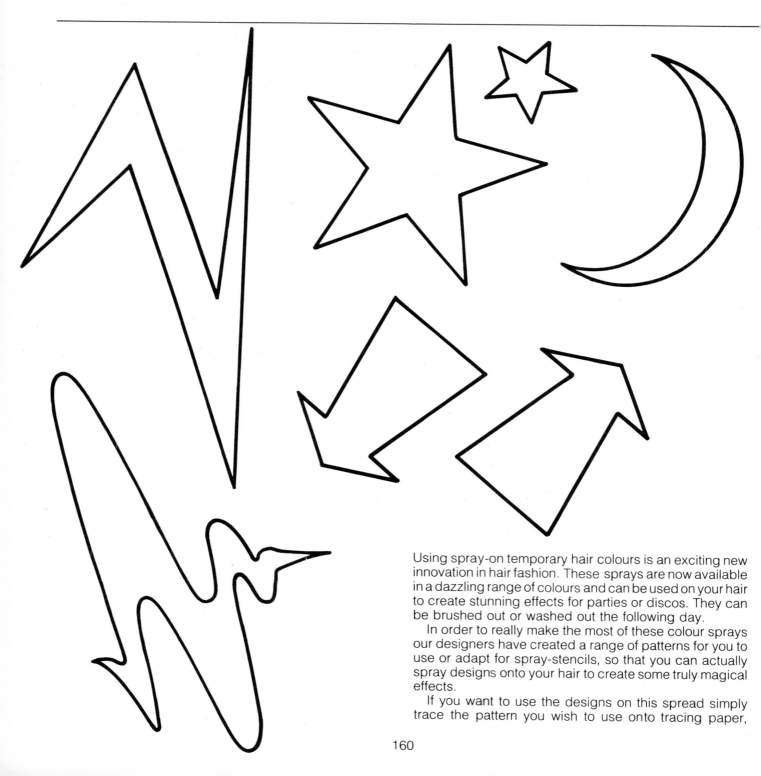

Using spray-on temporary hair colours is an exciting new innovation in hair fashion. These sprays are now available in a dazzling range of colours and can be used on your hair to create stunning effects for parties or discos. They can be brushed out or washed out the following day.

In order to really make the most of these colour sprays our designers have created a range of patterns for you to use or adapt for spray-stencils, so that you can actually spray designs onto your hair to create some truly magical effects.

If you want to use the designs on this spread simply trace the pattern you wish to use onto tracing paper,

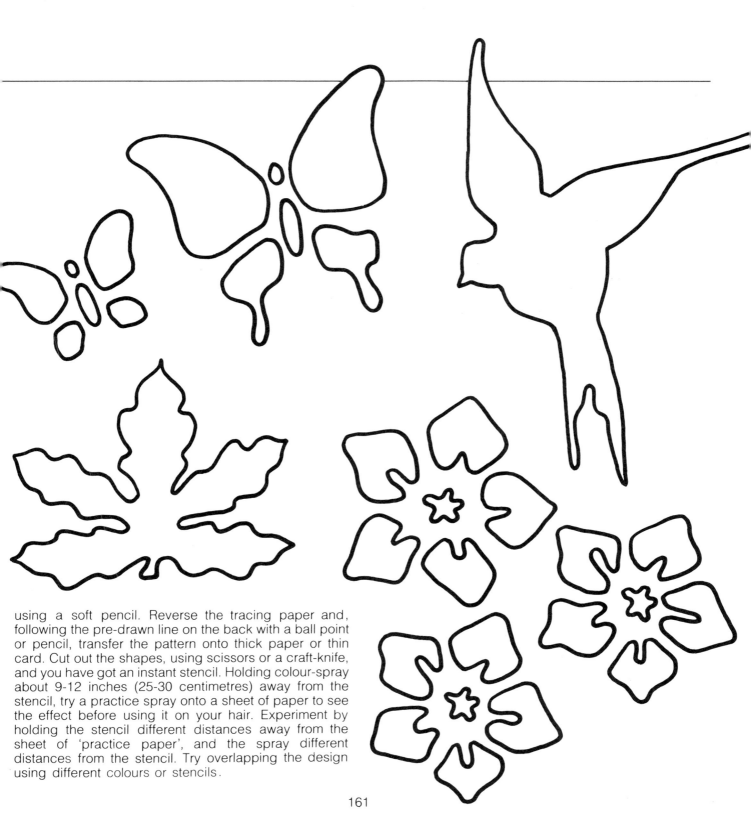

using a soft pencil. Reverse the tracing paper and, following the pre-drawn line on the back with a ball point or pencil, transfer the pattern onto thick paper or thin card. Cut out the shapes, using scissors or a craft-knife, and you have got an instant stencil. Holding colour-spray about 9-12 inches (25-30 centimetres) away from the stencil, try a practice spray onto a sheet of paper to see the effect before using it on your hair. Experiment by holding the stencil different distances away from the sheet of 'practice paper', and the spray different distances from the stencil. Try overlapping the design using different colours or stencils.

An A-Z of hair problems

Below you will find an A–Z of hair problems, their definitions, symptoms and possible remedies. However, if you do suspect that you have any of the following conditions consult a doctor or trichologist as soon as possible.

Alopecia

The Latin name for baldness – *alopecia* – is used by trichologists to describe many different types of hair loss. When the hair is lost in patches, the condition is known as *alopecia areata*; *alopecia totalis* is the term for total loss of hair on the head; and when there is total loss of hair all over the body the condition is known as *alopecia universalis*.

There are many reasons for hair loss. The condition may be due to illness or medical treatment. Medication with steroids, such as hydrocortisone in the treatment of inflamatory diseases and radiotherapy and chemotherapy used to treat cancer may well cause the hair to fall out. Stress, shock and inappropriate hairdressing treatments are other factors.

A poor diet, vitamin deficiency and anaemia are also frequently blamed for hair loss, and women often experience some hair loss both during and after pregnancy. However, once the problem has been identified and remedied, the hair growth usually returns to normal within a few months. Often an adequate diet may have to be combined with vitamin and mineral supplements. The B and C vitamins are thought to be most beneficial to hair growth together with zinc, iron and sulphur minerals.

Dandruff or scurf

Dandruff or scurf is a very common condition with people of all ages and both sexes. It is not usually an indication of poor health, but can be very annoying – especially when flakes appear on shoulders – and it is often very difficult to get rid of.

In those affected by dandruff, the outer layers of the epidermis of the scalp are shed unusually often and in relatively large scales which are easily seen. In most cases, however, dandruff is the result of a disorder of the sebaceous glands affecting the amount of sebum produced, known as seborrhoeic eczema. This can affect many parts of the skin apart from the scalp and is probably inherited. Another cause is psoriasis which is where production of new skin is speeded up and as a result its surface hardening does not take place. It is most common between the ages of 10 and 30.

Treatment usually consists of using anti-dandruff shampoos, which contain ingredients that remove the loose keratin scales from the scalp so that they are washed away. It will probably be necessary to use these shampoos at least twice a week at first. There are a great many on the market and it is important to make sure that you find the one that suits you best and then to stick with it. If fungi and bacteria are associated with the dandruff, a shampoo containing an antiseptic may be useful. A doctor or trichologist should be consulted if the condition persists or gets worse after several weeks of home treatment. For an over-dry scalp, an application of vitamin E oil as a hair tonic, which is allowed to soak in for at least half an hour, can be beneficial. For greasy hair and scalp, a dry shampoo, using bran, rubbed thoroughly through the scalp and then brushed out, has been proved to be very helpful.

If the shampoo has not been sufficiently rinsed away, it is easy to mistake the crusty deposits on the scalp for dandruff. It is worth trying out the following test: rub the scalp with a pad of cotton wool soaked in alcohol. After allowing the hair to dry, it should be brushed thoroughly. Massage the scalp and then carefully rinse the hair without using a shampoo; if the skin deposits are removed by the process then you do not have dandruff.

As dandruff is not an infection, it is unlikely that using anti-dandruff shampoo will cause the condition to cease. Anti-dandruff shampoos cannot cure the condition, only make it better temporarily. This is why it may be necessary to use these particular types of shampoo over a considerable period of time.

It may also be necessary to have frequent conditioning treatments when using an anti-dandruff shampoo.

Dermatitis

Dermatitis or eczema is usually caused by an allergy or skin irritant, although it is sometimes thought to be inherited. It can be associated with bacterial infection or nervous tension, and may cause severe itching. If the scalp is affected, a doctor should be consulted.

Anti-dandruff shampoos can sometimes be the answer, however, in many instances a very mild shampoo is found to be much more effective. In addition, care should be taken to improve general health; a vitamin B supplement can be beneficial.

Favus

Favus is a form of ringworm caused by the scalp being infected by a fungus. (See also ringworm on p. 165.)

Hair breakage

Hair breakage is very common if you are in poor health, in which case the hair splits and breaks until only a short stub remains. Hair can also break when chemicals used in various processes – for example, in bleaching or permanent waving – affect the hair adversely.

The harmful processes should be discontinued as soon as the cause is identified. Follow-up treatment should include applications of bland oils and hair conditioners.

Ichthyosis

Ichthyosis is a rare condition which is not confined to the scalp but may appear anywhere on the body. Most commonly found in very young children around two or three years old, it is a common hereditary disease and frequently occurs with several members of the same family. It is, however, not contagious and usually improves during adolescence.

With ichthyosis on the scalp, although the hair is usually normal at birth, later it will grow dull and scanty, especially on the top of the head. Thick, grey or brown scales will be seen on the crown of the scalp.

Although the scaliness may improve with treatment or age, a complete cure is usually very difficult to achieve. A supplement of vitamin A, plenty of sunshine and various creams can be beneficial.

It is important to remember that the person affected is usually highly sensitive to chemicals as well as being prone to skin infections.

Impetigo

This is a contagious condition caused by bacterial infection of the skin. It usually affects the areas around the mouth and nose but can affect the scalp.

The symptoms are small blisters which break showing moist red skin which develops a golden crust. It is most common among children and although not serious you should see a doctor. Hygiene is important to prevent the infection of others.

Lice

An infestation of lice can cause severe irritation to the scalp, and this may result in intense itching which can sometimes produce a secondary infection such as impetigo through the breaks in the skin resulting from constant scratching.

Lice are transmitted through close contact with those infected. They cannot be transmitted any other way as the lice can only survive a short time away from the body.

The female of the species lays her eggs on the hair close to the scalp. These eggs, known as nits, are grey coloured and, when laid, are glued to the surface of hair near the scalp.

It is to be hoped that treatment with an astringent lotion and/or a special shampoo will kill both lice and nits. However, even though dead, the nits remain stuck to the hairs on the head and are usually impossible to remove with ordinary brushes or combs. A fine metal comb, together with a special shampoo treatment, is needed to remove them. It is very difficult to make sure that all the nits are dead and to remove them all. Special care should be taken to check that the head is completely free from these pests. The nits are very small and are very difficult to see – especially if the hair is blond or light brown. If possible, each hair on the head should be examined – hence the phrase 'nit picking'.

Contrary to general opinion, lice are not attracted to really dirty hair. They actually prefer a clean head. So don't worry too much if you or, more likely, your children are suddenly infested. Unfortunately, there is still a social stigma attached to people suffering from this condition. It may be very upsetting to a young child who may not understand what is wrong. In this case it is best, when talking about the problem, to treat the matter as casually as possible.

All people who are in close contact with the individual affected should use the special shampoo, even though they themselves may not suffer from the complaint. It is also necessary to wash all clothing worn and bedding every day and to use a fumigant prior to laundering to prevent reinfection.

If a secondary infection has occurred, a doctor should be consulted. Anti-parasitic or antibiotic preparations are then usually given. These are likely to contain an insecticide and should be applied to the roots of the hair for several days.

Lichen Planus

This is a skin rash which can affect any part of the body. The condition causes itching and shows as small, violet, shiny spots. If it occurs on the scalp it can cause hair loss as it damages the hair follicles. This is a rare condition which usually affects the middle-aged. It is harmless but you should visit your doctor who will probably treat it with steroids to help the rash.

Mild hair loss

There are countless reasons for mild hair loss, including illness, a recent pregnancy, inadequate diet and vitamin or mineral deficiencies. In most cases, when the cause is eliminated, the hair loss will prove to be temporary and there is no cause for alarm. The ends of the hair often provide the clue as to the reason for the hair loss: if the ends taper to a point, this means the hairs are new; when they are frayed or blunt, they have broken off very close to the scalp, often as a result of chemical damage such as bleaching or perming.

As hair growth depends on good health, a balanced diet is essential. Supplements such as vitamin E, together with wheat germ and brewer's yeast, taken after meals, can help greatly to restore hair growth and good condition.

Neurodermatitis

Severe itching is one symptom of this relatively common condition, which starts as a red-based, scaly patch at the nape of the neck and at the hair margin. It frequently spreads to the adjoining skin and extends upwards under the hair. Although some hairs may be broken off at skin-level around the affected area, this is due to scratching rather than to the disease itself which does not immediately cause hair loss. Neurodermatitis is associated with mental tension. Someone who is tense tends to scratch and this, in turn, causes the habitual red, scaly patches of the disease.

Special lotions and creams can give relief. Sometimes the affected area is covered over with a plaster in order to break the scratching habit.

Odour

Hygiene is an important factor in hair care, not least because hair, being porous, tends to absorb any agent with which it comes into contact. You need only spend a relatively short time in a smoke-filled room and then emerge to realize just how strongly the smell of cigarette and cigar smoke can permeate your hair and clothes. It is also easy to forget that sweat glands exist all over the body, including the scalp. Although perspiration in itself is almost odourless, the bacteria that live in the secretion can accumulate and may frequently cause unpleasant smells.

Frequent shampooing is the only effective remedy, and regular conditioning which helps to protect the hair from pollution.

Oiliness

Oily hair is often a problem that first manifests itself at the change-over from puberty to adolescence. This is when, because of glandular and hormonal changes, the sebaceous glands become more active. When the oiliness is so acute that the hair looks as though it has been treated with an oily hair preparation, the condition is described as *seborrhoea*. When this happens, the hair looks limp with grease, even only one day after being washed. Sometimes infection sets in, causing hair loss. In some cases, scalps show an excessive degree of oiliness throughout life, although no disease is present.

In many instances, unfortunately, constant shampooing appears to make the condition worse rather than better. Professional advice should be sought from a doctor or trichologist if infection is present. A dry shampoo may be useful although these cannot be relied on indefinitely, and careful attention to diet, including limiting the intake of fatty foods and alcohol, can help. Exercise and plenty of fresh air will improve the skin tone and minimize the oiliness.

Psoriasis

Psoriasis manifests itself as thick and hard, dry silver scales which can appear almost anywhere on the body, including the scalp. The scales have a narrow, dark-red border just visible below and around the area of heaped-up scales. It is thought to be a hereditary condition. In uncomplicated cases, there is no itching or hair loss and the condition is not contagious. Severe crusting may occur and, although the skin may heal, the condition will recur throughout life.

Coal tar and other ointments can be helpful, but messy. Steroid creams and ultra-violet light treatments can be highly effective but they carry the risk of side effects.

Ringworm

The condition of ringworm is caused by fungi which invade the epidermis, or outermost layers of the scalp, and the hair shafts. It is highly contagious and at one time was a serious health problem in schools, reaching epidemic proportions. Many of these fungi have adapted to living on epidermal tissues, and are passed through direct contact or on dirty combs or clothing. There are many types of fungi which can be transmitted by shared hats, towels, pillows, brushes or combs. Patchy 'baldness', broken hairs and itchy scaling are all symptoms of ringworm and can occur singly or in combination. The patches, which can easily be seen, are not really bald but in fact consist of broken stumpy hairs.

A doctor will prescribe an antifungal agent which should be taken for one or two months until the fungus is fully eliminated. It most frequently affects children and can be caught from pets. In order to prevent reinfection, brushes and combs should be replaced and bed-linen should be washed thoroughly. The scalp and hair should

return to normal when the fungus has died off.

(See also favus on p. 163.)

Scalp allergies

Scalp allergies can be caused by virtually any substance, from food to the ingredients of hair dyes, shampoos and perfumes. This is why, for example, hair dyes should always be tested on a small area before being applied to the entire scalp. An allergic reaction to a substance can induce dermatitis (inflamation), which shows as a rash, swelling, blisters, or even oozing of the skin on the face, neck or scalp.

The first priority is to try to identify, if possible, the substance to which you are allergic. Once this has been identified and eliminated, theoretically the allergy should disappear completely. Often antihistamine drugs are prescribed in order to neutralize the allergic reaction.

Split ends

The use of strong chemicals, hot hair drying methods and environmental conditions such as exposure to sunlight can often have a degenerating effect on the hair, causing it to become very dry and brittle. If this happens, the ends may split and unfortunately there is no treatment available to make the hair knit together again.

The split ends should be trimmed and care should be taken to keep the hair shafts in good condition by avoiding harsh treatment.

Trichotillomania

Trichotillomania is a rare nervous condition which causes the person suffering from it to pull at the hair to such an extent that a bald patch is produced. Usually, the skin is normal and the few hairs that are left are quite short. The patch is usually irregularly shaped and often situated behind the ear or on the temples. Both adults and children can be affected and in some cases the habit begins by constant scratching of an area that is irritating.

Anyone affected by this condition should go to his or her doctor who will advise on treatment.

Index

Acknowledgements

Swallow Books gratefully acknowledge the assistance given to them in the production of *Hair Magic* by the following organizations and salons. We apologize to anyone we may have omitted to mention.

Photographs by:
John Andow 87, 108, 109, 131L B; H: Christine Harvey, Through the Looking Glass; MU: Leilani Kamen
Brian Marshall Photography Ltd 2, 3, 24L, 30, 31, 60, 61, 80, 81, 96 and 154

Illustrations by:
Coral Mula 26, 34, 35, 37, 43, 44, 45, 46, 47, 54, 55, 56, 57, 62, 63, 65, 83, 84, 85, 90, 100, 104, 105, 114, 115, 116, 117, 118, 126, 136
David Gifford 16, 17
Gerard Browne 38, 74
Prue Theobalds 78, 79

Alan International Hairdressing Salons 51, 95L; David Barron 66 P: Inter Salon Photography; Carole & Tony Bennett 35, 36, 40; Boots 18, 124; Braun 48T, 48B, 49T, 49M; British Caledonian 110; Camera Press 138, 140T, 140B, 141; Clipso (Watford & Hemel Hempstead) 6, 77L, 84B, 85, 117, 119L, 120L, 126, 127L, 128R, 153; Mary Evans Picture Library 10, 14R, 15T, 15B, 68L, 68TR, 121L, 121R, 143; Floridan 136T, 136B, 137, 144L, 144R, 145L, 146; The Fotomas Index 14L; John Frieda 58R; Joshua & Daniel Galvin 73 – H: Ivy, Colour: John, MU: Nigel at Sessions, P: Tony Boase, 90 – H: Ivy, Colour: John, MU: Nigel at Sessions P: Tony Boase 132; Sally & Richard Greenhill 20T; Harley Dean & Associates Ltd 148L, 148R; Henna Hair Health 44 – H: Neville Daniel; Johnson & Johnson Ltd 9L; Klorane 63L – P: Patrick Lichfield; Lâncome 33; L'Oreal 8R, 9R – H: Ranjit at Crimpers MU: Christine Saunders P: Al MacDonald, 43, 58M – H & MU: Tosh Reynolds, P: Al MacDonald, 59M – H: Bob Richardson, P: Alistair Hughes, 64TR – P: Al MacDonald, 77M – H: Shaun at Daniel Galvin, P: Alistair Hughes, 88L – H: Annette Town, P: Alistair Hughes, 95R – H: Stephen Way, 100, 101T – H: Bob Richardson for James Kimber, MU: Carol Langbridge for Dior, P: Adrien Feebig, 101B, 105 – P: Al MacDonald, 106 – H: Alan Stewart, Rainbow Rooms, 112R – H: Rita Rusk MU: Celia Hunter P: Al MacDonald; 119R – H: Bastian of Schumi, MU: Patti Burns P: Al MacDonald, 122L – H & MU: Tosh Reynolds P: Al MacDonald, 127R – H: Bastian at Schumi, P: Al MacDonald, 129 – H: Bastian at Schumi, MU: Patti Burns, P: Al MacDonald, 130 – MU: Celia Hunter, P: Al MacDonald, 133T, MU: Christine Saunders P: Al MacDonald, 135T – H: Howard at Toni & Guy, MU: Tosh Reynolds, P: Al MacDonald; Kevin Michael 77R, 122T; Michaeljohn 58L – H: Elliot, P: Al MacDonald, 64BR; Mothercare 37; Ocean Boulevard 24L, 39, 92, 120R, 125T; Phountzi 8L P: Michael Daks, Studio Phountzi; Pronuptia 134; Schumi 42, 71, 103, 114, 115, 116T; Schwarzkopf Ltd 50L, 50R, 64L, 76; Scruples 135B; Sherman Peru 89R – MU: Gilda, P: Daniel, 112L – MU: Tosh Reynolds, P: Mike Prior, 123 – MU: Tosh Reynolds, P: Mike Prior, 125B – MU: Helen Whiting, P: Phil Ward, 151 – MU: Tosh Reynolds, P: Mike Prior; Allan Soh 84T, 88R, 89L, 102; Philip Somerville 133B MU: Gilda White P: Eammon McCabe; Spectrum Colour Library 12, 13TL, 13BL, 20B, 22, 23, 26, 27, 29 122BR; Splinters International Ltd 99; Sporting Pictures (UK) Ltd 68BR, 111B; St. Clair's 69, 150 – MU: Theo for Flori Roberts ; Stanlee of Paris 145TR, 145B; Clifford Stafford 47, 49B – H: Carmel, P: Adrian Fibie, 62, 94 – P: Peter Brown, 113, 118 – H: Carmel, P: Peter Brown, 128L; Tony Stone Associates Ltd 13R, 131T; Warner Lambert 45 – H: Beverly Cobella MU: Patti Burris, P: Kenneth Bieber, 112M – H: Dar, MU: Nigel Plummer, P: Kenneth Bieber, 111T, 116B – H: Gregory, MU: Carol Langbridge, P: Kenneth Bieber, Stephen Way 59R, Courtesy of Wella Hair Cosmetics 19L, 19R, 52 H: Michael of Michaeljohn, MU: Celia Hunter, P: Al MacDonald; David Young 67.

L: Left R: Right M: Middle T: Top B: Bottom

H: Hair MU: Make-up P: Photographer

Our special thanks go to Christine Harvey of Through the Looking Glass, Fiona MacKilroy at L'Oreal and Nikki at Sherman Peru.